Monitoring, Birth Defects and Environment

THE PROBLEM OF SURVEILLANCE

Proceedings of a Symposium on
Monitoring, Birth Defects and Environment
Sponsored by the Birth Defects Institute
of the New York State Department of Health
Held at Albany, New York
October 19-20, 1970

Monitoring, Birth Defects and Environment
THE PROBLEM OF SURVEILLANCE

Edited by

Ernest B. Hook · Dwight T. Janerich · Ian H. Porter

Assistant Editors

Sally Kelly · Richard G. Skalko

Birth Defects Institute
New York State Department of Health
Albany, New York

ACADEMIC PRESS   NEW YORK AND LONDON   1971

ACADEMIC PRESS, INC.
111 Fifth Avenue, New York, New York 10003

United Kingdom Edition published by
ACADEMIC PRESS, INC. (LONDON) LTD.
24/28 Oval Road, London NW1 7DD

LIBRARY OF CONGRESS CATALOG CARD NUMBER: 70-179925

PRINTED IN THE UNITED STATES OF AMERICA

CONTENTS

I. INTRODUCTION

II. PRENATAL MONITORING

III. MONITORING MAJOR MALFORMATIONS

A. General Considerations

B. Specific Approaches

CONTENTS

IV. MONITORING MINOR MALFORMATIONS

A. Gross Defects

B. Dermatoglyphics

V. MONITORING MUTATIONS

A. Biochemical Approaches to Germinal Mutations

B. Biochemical Approaches to Somatic Mutations

PARTICIPANTS

Philip Banister, Child and Maternal Health Division, Department of National Health and Welfare, Ottawa, Ontario, Canada

Arthur D. Bloom, Department of Human Genetics, University of Michigan, Ann Arbor, Michigan

Maimon M. Cohen, Department of Pediatrics, State University of New York, Buffalo, New York

Allan J. Ebbin, Department of Pediatrics, University of Southern California Medical Center, Los Angeles, California

J. William Flynt, Jr., Epidemiology Program, Center for Disease Control, Atlanta, Georgia

F. C. Fraser, Department of Biology, McGill University, Montreal, Quebec, Canada

Alan M. Gittelsohn, Department of Biostatistics, Johns Hopkins University School of Hygiene and Public Health, Baltimore, Maryland

Kurt Hirschhorn, Department of Pediatrics, Mt. Sinai School of Medicine, New York, New York

Ernest B. Hook, Birth Defects Institute, New York State Department of Health, Albany, New York

Dwight T. Janerich, Birth Defects Institute, New York State Department of Health, Albany, New York

Sally Kelly, Birth Defects Institute, New York State Department of Health, Albany, New York

Samuel Milham, Jr., Washington State Department of Health and Social Services, Olympia, Washington

James R. Miller, Department of Paediatrics, University of British Columbia School of Medicine, Vancouver, British Columbia

Robert W. Miller, Epidemiology Branch, National Cancer Institute, Bethesda, Maryland

Edmond A. Murphy, Department of Medicine, Johns Hopkins University School of Medicine, Baltimore, Maryland

Ian H. Porter, Birth Defects Institute, New York State Department of Health, Albany, New York

I. Herbert Scheinberg, Department of Medicine, Albert Einstein College of Medicine, Bronx, New York

Thomas H. Shepard, Department of Pediatrics, University of Washington School of Medicine, Seattle, Washington

Richard G. Skalko, Birth Defects Institute, New York State Department of Health, Albany, New York

David W. Smith, Department of Pediatrics, University of Washington School of Medicine, Seattle, Washington

H. Eldon Sutton, Department of Zoology, University of Texas, Austin, Texas

Lowell Weitkamp, Department of Anatomy, University of Rochester School of Medicine and Dentistry, Rochester, New York

FOREWORD

This volume is the record of a Symposium held in Albany, New York on October 19 and 20, 1970, sponsored by the Birth Defects Institute of the New York State Department of Health.

Such a Symposium is in keeping with the tradition of the Department's long history of dedication to the advancement and dissemination of scientific knowledge in order to meet the ever changing challenges to our people's health. Our first research endeavors began in the 1890's, were supplemented in 1914 with the establishment of the Division of Laboratories and Research, and they have continued to expand ever since. We have devoted a significant fraction of our operating funds to supporting and carrying out all manner of research, ranging from cancer research at our Roswell Park Memorial Institute to research in kidney disease under the auspices of our Kidney Disease Institute.

The Birth Defects Institute has existed for only three years and I think it has already accomplished much—for the patient, in education, and at the laboratory bench, all in the service of the people of the State of New York. It has established several units concerned with the critical aspect of the problem of birth defects; these include laboratories, population investigation units, genetic counseling clinics which provide help for families and physicians, and a Birth Defects Information Service.

This Symposium was the Institute's first such scientific gathering. The comprehensive program is an example of the Institute's forward-going approach to the critical questions to which we are seeking answers. These are as broad and extensive as the future of man and are as finite and immediate as our children's health. Indeed, the problems and methods examined in this volume could not be centered in a more critical area than the environment and its influence on heredity and birth defects. To generate and exchange these ideas, the Institute brought together a distinguished group of scientists whose deliberations are presented here.

Hollis S. Ingraham, M.D.
Commissioner
New York State Department of Health
Albany, New York

ACKNOWLEDGMENTS

The meeting upon which this volume is based could not have taken place without the expert administrative efforts of Edwin C. Jones and Sylvia Sickles. To them, and the rest of the staff of the Birth Defects Institute, and to Ellen Heenehan for her assistance in the preparation and typing of the final manuscript, we express our thanks and appreciation.

EDITORS' NOTE

The reader will note inconsistencies between chapters in matters of style, particularly with regard to citations. Since the gestation of this volume was unduly prolonged (by matters over which the editors, publishers, and authors had no control), we elected to present the material in its present form rather than further delay the appearance of the volume in order to achieve stylistic homogeneity. The reader will judge for himself whether any of these inconsistencies represent "variants" or "defects," major or minor.

I. INTRODUCTION

GENERAL INTRODUCTION

The goal of surveillance as considered in this volume is to monitor the incidence of malformations and mutations in the population to detect the introduction or the increase of unsuspected mutagens and teratogens in the environment.

Population monitoring is clearly an indirect and difficult way of detecting environmental hazards. But obvious ethical and practical limitations preclude attempts to investigate human mutagenic and teratogenic effects directly. And despite recent progress in experimental teratology and mutagenesis it still appears a long way off before all environmental agents to which we are exposed can be investigated by approaches in the laboratory that are both ethically acceptable and clinically relevant.

Thus, while monitoring is not the definitive method of investigating human teratogens and mutagens, it still may be the most practical way to detect and eventually limit the effects of such agents.

The outstanding question is the choice of marker(s) to be monitored. The Symposium upon which this volume is based was called to consider the particular advantages, difficulties and possible refinements of potential marker systems for teratogens and mutagens.

The methods described for surveillance of major birth defects and/or fetal wastage as markers are rough systems, but ready ones, which can be progressively refined with time and relatively little money. Their main advantage is their low cost, since in most cases they use records (or specimens) already collected for other purposes. Their main disadvantages are the difficulties with ascertainment and our ignorance of how to analyze data involving different types of defects or wastage. In an initial analysis, for example, should we distinguish types of t. e. fistulas or pool all gastrointestinal malformations together? We may not be able to answer such questions until after additional human teratogens have been identified, but the purpose of surveillance is to detect hitherto unknown teratogens, not study the effects of known ones.

It is likely to be a much more formidable task to monitor the effects of teratogenic agents whose action on the fetus is not apparent until long after birth. The extent of preventable prenatal "environmental" causes of mental retardation, learning disorders, psychological maladjustment and cerebral palsy remain unknown. It is an open question whether monitoring for indirect markers detectable in the neonate, such as minor birth defects or low birth weight, will be sensitive to such agents.

Separate problems exist in monitoring point mutations manifested by protein changes. But one advantage of this approach is that, in the first analysis at least, we can pool events from many different systems. Even if agents differ in their mode of action they are not likely to be locus specific. More elaborate techniques are required for monitoring mutations, however, and the costs are much higher. Of course, these would be a cheap price to pay if accurate ascertainment of mutations would eventually lead to their reduction. Unfortunately, greater knowledge of the distribution of the human mutation rate in time and space does not guarantee that a practical application can be made of this information <u>post hoc</u>. The same is true of accurate ascertainment of major defects and fetal wastage. A great deal is known about the population variables associated with the occurrence of anencephaly, for instance, but this has not yet led to discovery and abatement of contributing environmental factors. The likelihood of identifying a presumed environmental cause of a future increase in any marker appears moot.

Nevertheless, these questions are too important to ignore because cheap or complete methods are not yet available. If teratogenic or mutation rates are increasing, then this problem merits the investment of society's resources. And if they are not, the costs of surveillance may still be justified if only to determine that fact. Clearly these questions are propitious and merit our attention.

WHY MONITOR?[*]

Edmond A. Murphy

The main activity of medicine is monitoring in one form or another: what defines the scope of the present Symposium is that it deals with the effects of vigilance at the very start of life. If this is not to be mere idle curiosity, the emphasis must be on the word "effects". When begins my ditty.

We start, I think with three questions. What are we hoping to observe? Does it throw any light on causative relationships? What are we to do about it?

What are we hoping to observe?

There are always observations to be made. Whether they are useful depends on two things: first coherence which implies that a pattern exists on which the observations may bear; second the resolving power of analysis which will ensure that the pattern is not lost in noise.

There is little information as to how efficient monitoring is. We may know harmful factors which have been discovered, but have no idea how many may have been missed. In face of this, something is to be learned about strategy in monitoring from considering a few of the outstanding examples of successful detection.

The following points I think can be substantiated.

[*]Paper #471 from the Department of Biostatistics, Johns Hopkins University School of Public Health.

1. Directed searches are more likely to be
fruitful than undirected. It is unfortunate but
true that the common practice in teaching is to
play up the value of the fortuitous -- the fungus
contaminating the Petri dish or the train stop-
ping beside some particolored sheep -- as a
source for scientific advancement and to gloss
over the large number of such observations which
have been followed up without reward. Who knows
how much misdirection of effort this has led to?
The classical studies by which Muller (1) demonstrated the mutagenic effects of X-rays in
Drosophila were not undertaken as part of a vague
unfocused survey of factors which might be of
value in experimental mutagenesis. As Muller
points out there were already numerous reports
in the literature that exposure to X-rays leads
to defective development of the embryo but they
were so vague as to throw little light on patho-
genesis.

2. Many discoveries are fortuitous. Then the
gross change will be detected more easily than
the minor; the bizarre than the commonplace; the
immediate than the remote. The prompt recognition from three apparently independent sources
(2-4) of the teratogenic effects of thalidomide
admirably illustrates these points. The abnormalities were certainly gross and ordinarily rare;
and they appeared within a few months of the
existing cause. But had the effects of
thalidomide been to produce a 20% increase in
duodenal ulcers in the offspring twenty years or
so later, the ill effects might have been just as
great or greater and therefore just as important
to prevent. But how easily would the relationship of cause to effect have been detected?
Not the least of the difficulties would be the
scattering in time and in space after such a long
incubation period. Yet perhaps long term common-

place effects may be the usual pattern though one which we may be almost powerless to detect.

3. Results in monitoring are to be obtained by a punctilious attention to both the cases observed and to the population from which they have been observed. The first report on rubella as a teratogen came from Gregg (5) an ophthalmologist who was impressed not so much by the increased frequency of congenital cataract as that it was of an unusual type. An epidemiologist concerned primarily with frequency of congenital cataract in a population might very well have missed this point, just as, for example he might have lumped phocomelia due to thalidomide under "other congenital defects". Precision of diagnosis is a cardinal feature of monitoring.

4. It cannot be too strongly stated that the best use of the results is most likely to be obtained by a free communication among the basic scientist, the clinician and the epidemiologist. The rubella-cataract problem could be elucidated only because Gregg had access to two other pieces of information: that at the appropriate stage of pregnancy an unusually severe outbreak of rubella had occurred, information obtained by the epidemiologist, and that various infectious organisms could be transmitted across the placenta; information provided by the basic scientist. Finally, of course, the primary conclusions led to a search for other congenital defects with results which are now well known.

Again the first recognition of retrolental fibroplasia was of course clinical. Its sudden appearance as a disease, almost exclusively of the premature child, excited much discussion culminating in a conscientious but inconclusive survey and review of changes in the handling of such infants, by Kinsey and Zacharias (6). They

inculpated three possible factors: water-soluble
vitamins, iron and oxygen. Campbell (7) noted
that oxygen, in the premature, causes edema of
the feet apparently because of defective capillaries and she thought a similar mechanism might
be at work in the eyes. Her focusing of attention
on oxygen she attributes to undocumented rumors
presumably emanating from Crosse and Evans who
reported their results elsewhere (8-10). Evans
(9) in his paper, quotes the experimental studies
of Campbell on oxygen tension and the growth of
capillaries in the eye (11).

5. Monitoring is perhaps directed too much
to detecting and explaining abnormal increases
above background. But the "background" cases
themselves may be due to some factor for which we
should be monitoring. For instance there is
little concern expressed about chromosomal non-
disjunctions except in relationship to drugs.
But the habitual levels themselves must be examined, and a familiar approach is to look for
clustering in space or time. Clustering in space
may be hard to establish because of varying
diagnostic standards. But clustering in time
show up.

Since virus infections are seasonal it might be
supposed that nondisjunction might, with an appropriate time lapse, also be seasonal. Robinson
and Puck (12) have explored whether nondisjunc-
tions exhibit seasonal clustering and the results
remain tentative. If such a pattern is difficult
to demonstrate on close scrutiny then it is
unlikely to be recognized on casual inspection.

The persistence with which a pattern is pursued
depends on prior considerations, not all of them
scientific. I suspect, for instance, that the
energy which has been lavished on exploring the
side effects of hallucinogenic drugs has, as much
as anything else, been political.

Does it throw any light on causative relationships?
There is a wide gulf between the inferences
from deliberate experimentation and from data
generated by the spontaneous behavior of populations, however carefully observed. Ethical and
other considerations commonly preclude experimentation in man. Data from animal experiments,
however, are often of doubtful relevancy. Genetics owes a great debt to the study of mice,
Drosophila and bacteria: but to apply wholesale
the findings from these species to medicine
would be hazardous.

The very word "monitor" implies that we observe
but do not manipulate. This limitation seems
inescapable in man though perhaps we can make
inroads upon it, for example, by the study of
tissue culture. But the inferences are weak.
The effects of LSD on chromosome breaks in man in
vivo may not be explorable by direct experimentation; but in data from populations taking this
drug of their own accord the effects will be
confounded with those of other mechanisms. Perhaps people who use LSD are on other drugs also
or suffer more from infectious diseases, or drink
more alcohol, or smoke more, or suffer more from
the ill-effects of long hair.

The possible scope for monitoring is immense.
There are two approaches. In the a priori method
every new physical procedure or chemical is
tested for its ill-effects. In such a vast under-
taking duplication of effort may be minimized by
exploiting whatever equivalences there may be
between carcinogenesis, mutagenesis and teratogenesis. The a posteriori method is to wait for
anomalies to occur and then to trace them to their
sources.

The problem of demonstrating an effect involves
resolution from a scientific, and power from a
statistical, standpoint.

Scientifically the more immediately the data is related to the phenomena of interest, the better. In genetic terms, for instance, the closer the measurement to the site of gene action the better as Penrose (13) demonstrated admirably in a classical paper. From a statistical standpoint, a continuous treatment of variables is more powerful than a categorical one. For example, we learn more by considering whether the number of chromosome breaks increases regularly with the dose of a drug than by comparing means in persons on the drug and those not on it. In general, the more explicit the model used in analysis the more powerful the tests and the more refined the conclusions. It seems hardly necessary to make this point at all except for the fact that it is surprisingly often overlooked.

The dangers of ignoring the denominator are, or should be, well known. A new clinic for birth defects would be at best a hazardous source of information about the prevalence of a disorder. If the clinic has a stable catchment, ascertainment of cases is complete, the racial and age composition of the population is not changing, and so forth, trends may be assessed from such a source with reasonable confidence. But since these conditions are usually not fulfilled, much finesse may be required from the epidemiologist.

Two major statistical problems arise in attempting to test for dependence. First, an ideal system of inference would require that we treat hypotheses symmetrically, perhaps introducing cost functions to take account of practicalities. Yet, it is not possible to pursue this course without using prior probabilities which are usually not known. Thus in practice we are driven to treat the comparison asymmetrically. We talk of the "onus of proof" supposing that radiation is harmless until proved otherwise, or harmful until proved otherwise. In the political supervision of chemical compounds there has been a gradual shift in emphasis from the one to the other.

Secondly, the statement that a drug has an effect "significant at the one percent level" means that if the drug is indeed inert there is a one percent chance of getting an effect as marked as this or more marked. If 1,000 inert drugs are tested we can expect ten of them to give results "significant" by this criterion. Now with therapeutic agents, subsequent experience will demonstrate the spuriousness of this conclusion. But if a significant result leads to prohibition of that drug, there would be no further experience.

I think that this problem arises because of an excessively empirical approach to monitoring. If statistics is made responsible for what is properly the domain of pharmacology or biochemistry, we can hardly blame it if it breaks down under the strain.

One other point for caution. I have said that observation leads to less cogent conclusions than experimentation. It is possible to demonstrate cause by the latter but rarely, perhaps never, by the former. From observation alone, we cannot empirically prove that the factors associated represent cause and effect. It is necessary to establish a rational connection between the putative cause and the effect, and to prove that eliminating the cause abolishes the effect. Thus, we have come full circle. The culminations of the epidemiological study must be a rationale which will come from the basic scientists, and the therapeutic or preventive intervention which will come from the clinicians, or sometimes, from those in public health.

What are we to do about it?

Information from monitoring might be used in the following ways:

(1) By modifying environmental factors to reduce the risks of point mutation, translocation, nondisjunction or defective ontogeny. Such steps include control of drugs and prevention of infections.

(2) For genetic traits already established, to identify those parents who have a high risk of defective progeny and persuade them not to have children.

(3) To modify the maternal-fetal interaction in such a way as to avoid disease in the fetus. Obvious examples would be the treatment of Rh incompatibility or maternal syphilis; and perhaps, though the data are less compelling (14), to treat maternal biochemical anomalies such as hyperphenylalaninemia or endocrine upset such as myxedema.

(4) Postnatal correction of the defect by special diet, by operation, by special schooling and so forth.

(5) As a last resort, by abortion of defective fetuses.

Which of these courses are adopted depends on a large number of factors -- medical, political, ethical, social, and moral -- many of which will arise in the course of the symposium.

But there is a wider issue. We must confront seriously the question of what our precise objectives may be and here it seems to me there are three major considerations.

First, there is distribution of the burden. In Diagram 1 is represented an elemental tension. Consider a genetic condition, such as muscular dystrophy, in a population of stable size where the homozygous wildtype is the fittest. It can be shown that ultimately the number of genetic deaths produced is, on the average, independent of the force of selection. A disorder such as the Duchenne type of muscular dystrophy which is lethal, in the long run produces no more genetic deaths than a mildly unfit X-linked recessive such as color-blindness. Any measure, then, which maintains unfit genes in the population has no effect ultimately on the number of deaths produced but merely redistributes the deaths. For example, hemophilia in a primitive society would probably be lethal so that the gene would become extinct in the male line in one generation. Where the males live long enough to reproduce, the harmful gene will be more widely scattered and instead of one family having many sons dying of this disorder, many families will be afflicted with children who are somewhat less fit, and who will have smaller families, and perhaps will die prematurely, though not necessarily in childhood. In general, then, the effect of therapeutics and (in the case of recessives) promotion of outbreeding is to shift the load from the individual family to the entire population. It is, if you like, similar to the spreading of liability by an insurance scheme. Conversely, inbreeding and eugenic measures shift the load in the opposite direction.

If no carriers of the sickle gene were to have children the gene would be eliminated in one generation. But it might be felt that this concentrates the penalty very unfairly. If heterozygotes married only homozygous wildtype people no children would have sickle cell disease and this would remove the heaviest burden from the family. Such a policy makes the heterozygous state more common.

Some theoretical calculations are presented in Table 1, for an autosomal recessive character, lethal in the homozygous state. The fitness of the heterozygote is arbitrary. The mutation rate is 10^{-5} and the back mutation rate 10^{-7}. For convenience all frequencies have been multiplied by 10^5. These are frequencies in the mating population after selection. The equilibrium frequency of the mutant under random mating is first computed. Then obligatory backcross mating is introduced, i.e. allowing heterozygotes to marry only persons homozygous for the normal gene. The frequencies of the mutant gene are computed 1, 5, and 20 generations later, and at equilibrium. It is only when the fitness of the heterozygote is close to unity that the policy has any substantial ultimate effect on gene frequency. If the fitness is 99% or less, the increase in gene frequency is less than 10%. The number of genetic deaths per generation is the same for all equilibrium states. If the fitness of the heterozygote is unity or greater there comes a stage at which there are more hetero- zygotes than homozygotes and the eugenic policy cannot be maintained.

I chose to consider genetic death to illustrate the point that in deciding on policy we must not be distracted by superficial successes. But, of course there is more to consider: the burden of impaired health, incapacity, frank illnesses and pain, and premature death.

The second consideration, however, is what kind of population we would like. Here a fundamental problem in epistemology arises. We, who make that decision, are part of the class of things to be selected and, therefore, prejudiced. Certainly we do not aim to produce more anence- phalic babies or children with phocomelia. But few decisions are so clear cut. It is by no means obvious whether or not we want big people or little people; whether unlimited intelligence is a desirable characteristic; or whether the schizoid personality has value. I do not subscribe to the view that the average is necessarily, either the normal or the optimal (15).

But apart from the desiderata in the individual we must also give thought to the desiderata in the population.

It is an old criticism, that if the criterion of fitness is survival of the species, the principle of the "survival of the fittest" reduces to the "survival of the survivors". But even fitness in the narrow sense of survival value is elusive. The practical criterion commonly used by the geneticist is the average number of progeny of completed families. But over what set of outcomes are we computing the average? Results over one or two generations may be misleading. To consider the family only and not the population may also mislead. Always the emphasis tends to be on averages because they are the easiest of the statistical moments to compute. But since the environment may change drastically and what may be an optimal genome for one state may not be optimal for another, in the long run variability in the gene pool is of the highest importance to the survival of the species. If eugenics were to eliminate the sickle gene, an important capacity for adaptation would be missing from the gene pool should falciparal malaria again become widespread.

A more refined system of adaptation to the "optimal" exists for multilocal characters. Moreover the more loci involved the smaller the scatter about the optimal. Thus the price paid for the preservation of the adaptability of the species, a heavy one in such single locus disorders as the hemoglobinopathies, is diminished. It would be a formidable task to eliminate such a multilocal system entirely, even in a fast-breeding laboratory animal. Whether we could do this at all in man is doubtful. But such tampering we would undertake at our peril.

Closely related to this is the third problem. If we could abolish mutations should we do so? Granted that evolution has progressed by the operation of selection on mutations, it seems evident that by abolishing mutation we will arrest evolution. It is certainly true, as every politician knows, that chaos is easier to create than order and that a new mutation is much more likely to be harmful than otherwise. But it might well be argued that averages have very little to do with progress and that avoidance of evil is a poor excuse for sacrificing the good. Who is to say how many deaths are a fair price to produce one Shakespeare?

CONCLUSION

Why monitor?

We monitor because there is some prospect that we may diminish the consequences of environmental indiscretions and do something to eliminate useless genetic mutations.

Effective monitoring will first demonstrate causal relationships and perhaps suggest remedies. Demonstration of causal relationships is not to be achieved by arrogant isolationism. The example of retrolental fibroplasia, surely one of the triumphs of monitoring, illustrates the joint need for clinical observation, epidemiological method and a reassuring rationalization of an empirial relationship by a demonstration of pertinent mechanisms.

For the rest, how we formulate policy when we understand the etiology is a serious issue to some facets of which I have called brief attention. There is nothing which should be so thoroughly questioned as the obvious.

REFERENCES

1. Muller, H.J., Artificial transmutation of the gene. Science 66 84-87, 1927.
2. Lenz, W. Kindliche Missbildungen nach Medikament-Ennahme während der Gravidität. Dtsch. med.Wsch. 86 2555, 1961.
3. Pfeiffer, R.A. and Kosnow, W., Zur Frage einer exogenen Verursachung von schweren Extremitätinmissbildungen. Munch. med. Wschr. 104 68, 1962.
4. McBride, W. G., Thalidomide and congenital anomalies. Letter to Lancet 1961 2 1358.
5. Gregg, N.M., Congenital cataract following German measles in the mother. Trans. Ophth. Soc. Aust. 3 35-46, 1941.
6. Kinsey, V.E. and Zacharias, L., Retrolental fibroplasia. Incidence in different localities in recent years and a correlation of the incidence with treatment given the infants. J. Amer. Med. Assoc. 139 572, 1949.
7. Campbell, K., Intensive oxygen therapy as a possible cause of retrolental fibroplasia: a clinical approach. Med. J. Aust. 1951 2 48.
8. Crosse, V.M., The problem of retrolental fibroplasia in the city of Birmingham. Trans. Ophthal. Soc. U.K. 71 609, 1951.
9. Evans, P.J., Retrolental fibroplasia. Trans. Ophthal. Soc. U.K. 71 613, 1951.
10. Crosse, V.M. and Evans, P.J., Prevention of retrolental fibroplasia. Arch. Ophth 48 83, 1952.
11. Campbell, F.W., The influence of a low atmospheric pressure on the development of the retinal vessels in the rat. Trans. Ophthal. Soc. U.K. 71 287, 1951.

12. Robinson, A. and Puck, T.T., Studies on chromosomal nondisjunction in man II. Am. J. Hum. Genet. 19 112, 1967
13. Penrose, L.S., An introduction to human biochemical genetics. Eugen. Lab. Memoirs XXXVII. Cambridge University Press, London, 1955.
14. Arthur, L.J.H. and Hulme, J.D., Intelligent, small for dates baby born to oligophrenic mother after low phenylaline diet during pregnancy. Pediatrics 46 235-239, 1970.
15. Murphy, E. A., A scientific viewpoint on normalcy. Perspect. Biol. Med. 9 333, 1966.

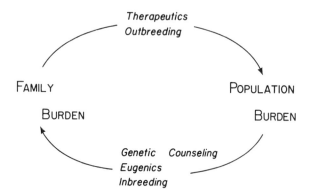

Figure 1. Factors affecting the distribution of the burden of genetic disorders.

Table 1

The effects of obligatory backcrossing on the frequency of an autosomal recessive lethal.
The mutation rate is arbitrarily set at 10^{-5} and the back mutation rate at 10^{-7}.

Fitness of the heterozygote	Equilibrium frequency with random mating $\times 10^5$	Gene frequency after indicated number of generations of backcross mating. $(\times 10^5)$			
		1	5	20	∞
0.8	7.998	7.999	7.999	8.000	8.000
0.9	17.984	17.985	17.990	17.997	17.998
0.95	37.857	37.864	37.888	37.944	37.993
0.99	181.499	181.662	182.298	184.466	197.804
0.999	538.765	540.211	545.980	567.406	1978.060
0.9999	620.592	622.512	630.187	658.935	18160.175
1.0000	630.451	632.432	640.356	670.061	*

* No equilibrium is attained since the heterozygotes become so numerous that there are insufficient homozygous partners for them.

II. PRENATAL MONITORING

THE POSSIBLE USE OF AMNIOCENTESIS FOR MONITORING

Kurt Hirschhorn

Perhaps the most promising method for monitoring in the future may be the use of amniocentesis. This requires the assumption that all symposia held recently on prenatal diagnosis and on amniocentesis will lead to some kind of a large population study in which either an unselected, or perhaps sooner, a selected group of pregnancies will be examined. For example, all pregnancies in mothers over forty years of age would provide us with a defined bias of selection. Everything discussed below is based on the assumption that such studies will occur. (I am not saying whether I favor or do not favor such studies, but from what has been said in the various symposia, there may be a reasonable chance that somewhere a pilot project will be begun, to monitor either selected groups of pregnant women, or perhaps there will even be universal monitoring in a few centers. `

Let me briefly review the technique that is used. One obtains a few ml. of amniotic fluid transabdominally. (In a recent symposium in New York, it was concluded that the risk of amniocentesis to mother and child is probably quite small.) After obtaining the fluid, one separates the fluid from the cellular components which are fetal in origin, although some evidence of maternal contamination has been found. One can then study the supernatant fluid for certain biochemical characteristics and one can study the cells either directly, by means of cytochemical and biochemical techniques, or one can culture the cells. These cultures can then be used for two purposes: (1) to produce chromosome preparations and (2) to do biochemical studies on the larger volume of cells obtained from the tissue culture.

What relevant information can be obtained for the purpose of monitoring? First, let us consider chromosomes. We can observe breaks and recombinations. The meaning of these and their relevance to monitoring is discussed by Cohen and Bloom elsewhere in this volume.

Perhaps more important are stable aberrations discovered prenatally, such as balanced or unbalanced translocations. The finding of such events in the fetus, in the presence of normal chromosomes in the parents is, of course, evidence for a new chromosomal mutation.

It is now possible to detect a number of biochemical diseases by means of prenatal diagnosis. The list is rapidly expanding but currently 27 different disorders can be monitored in utero. However, this is not a practical approach. Most of these disorders are autosomal recessives and one would, therefore, monitor for defects and not for new mutations. A more useful approach might use the many normal genetic polymorphisms of cellular enzymes. Some of these are common, that is, occur with a high gene frequency. Others are rare variants. There is now available an ever growing number of common polymorphisms, which are not important for our purpose, as well as the critical rare variants. These may, perhaps, be useful for the detection of mutation rates in man and could, of course, be monitored in cord blood. However, again assuming that we are going to monitor prenatally, one can detect these variants at a time when one has the parents available and observe whether the variant is a new mutation, that is, absent in the parents. The presence of the parents and the relatively short interval between conception and monitoring would also allow a more accurate exposure history. Therefore, if a large population is screened prenatally, this technique may provide the most accurate estimate of the current mutation rate and, in the future, of any changes in that rate.

COLLECTION OF HUMAN EMBRYOS AND FETUSES

A Centralized Laboratory for Collection
of Human Embryos and Fetuses:
Seven years Experience: I. Methods[1]

Thomas H. Shepard, M.D.
Thomas Nelson, M.D.[2]
Godfrey P. Oakley, Jr., M.D.[3]
Ronald J. Lemire, M.D.

1. Supported by grants from the National
    Institutes of Health (HD00836,
    5-T01-HD-00180 and DE02918).

2. Postdoctoral Research Trainee
    supported by grant 5-T01-HE0180 from
    the National Institutes of Health.

3. Supported by Department of Health,
    Education and Welfare, Public Health
    Services and Mental Health Administration
    Center for Disease Control.

OUTLINE

I.   Introduction

II.   Objectives

III.   Methods used in the collection
        Mechanics of initiation
        Source of specimens
        Method of delivery of specimens
        Cooperation of the obstetricians and
            pathologists
        Examination of specimens
        Costs

IV.   Teaching

V.   Research and utilization
        Number of specimens
        Number and type of investigators
            supplied
        Serial and sectioned specimens

VI.   Monitoring fetal and embryonic loss
        Advantages and example of use
        Problems
        Other uncontrolled variables
        Research without a hypothesis

VII.   Summary

INTRODUCTION

In the first of these two papers, we propose to
review some of our experiences and observations
with a laboratory for collection of human embryos
and fetuses. The collection was started seven
and a half years ago and now includes 1365 specimens. The original technics in most cases
evolved from observations of the methods of the
Carnegie Institution, Department of Embryology,
then in Baltimore, and from the Fetal Laboratory
in the Department of Human Anatomy, University of
Copenhagen. The laboratory is maintained by
pediatricians and although much sound advice has
been received from anatomists and obstetricians,
a recognized bias unfortunately exists because of
the lack of active participation by these two
disciplines. We propose to discuss in more
detail than previous reports[1-7] the technics of
procurement and utilization of specimens. Some
general comments on the use of the collection as
a monitoring system for defects are made.

II OBJECTIVES

Although not all the objectives were predeter-
mined at the start of the collection, they have
evolved into the following areas:

1. Teaching
2. Research and Utilization
3. Monitoring Fetal and Embryonic Loss

III METHODS USED IN COLLECTION

Mechanics of initiation. An advisory committee
for the collecting laboratory consisting of
persons interested in either procurement or utilization of specimens was formed. In our case,

professors of obstetrics, anatomy (embryology)
and genetics along with an active and respected
member of the practicing obstetrical community
served as a valuable source of advice on general
policies. One of the first problems was found to
be the presence of multiple investigators all
attempting to collect human fetal and embryonic
material; this problem was solved by indicating
to the other collectors that with a new centralized system the number and state of preservation
of their specimens would be increased. Relatively few of these persons were competing for
collection of the same organ; to our knowledge
the collecting system has been able to completely
satisfy these investigators. No other separate
collection has been initiated in the Seattle area
during the past seven years.

We chose two local hospitals at the start and
subsequently increased the number to four. The
hospital administrator, the head of obstetrics,
and the head of pathology were all visited
personally by the laboratory director and the
plans discussed. In most cases no objections
were found, but often a number of serious problems were obviated by thorough discussion.

Source of specimens. The four hospitals are
within a 15 minute drive from the laboratory.
Their combined obstetrical beds number 108 and
the yearly live-born deliveries are approximately
6,500. The percentage of available specimens
supplied to the laboratory varied widely between
hospitals and between obstetricians. No abrupt
attempts to increase the intake have been made;
the reasons for the variability of intake and our
relaxed attitude about it are discussed below
under item VI.

Some specimens from other hospitals or clinics
are accepted if they are of teaching or research
interest.

Methods of delivery of specimens. During the
daytime specimens are picked up by a laboratory
technician or in certain cases when the material
is especially valuable (i.e. therapeutic
abortion by hysterotomy or small well preserved
embryo) by a physician from the laboratory. When
indicated, one or several electron microscopists
may accompany a physician from the laboratory to
the operating room and obtain tissue within
minutes of delivery. At night if it seems likely
that a valuable specimen will be obtained, the
pick-up is performed by one of the investigators
from the laboratory. Both at night and in the
operating room, the physical presence of a laboratory investigator acts to demonstrate the value
of the material and allows the investigator to
advertise some merits of the collecting laboratory.

The centralization and continuity of collection
is a big help to referring obstetricians and
nurses; there is never any question about the
need for specimens, nor the place to telephone.
Specimens from the four regularly supplying
hospitals are always accepted; consequently the
form of material may vary from a few clots to the
body of a newborn. In the delivery rooms, operating rooms and emergency rooms there are a number of bottles labeled with the laboratory name,
instructions and telephone numbers (night or
daytime). The bottles contain no fixative; a
particularly important point due to the fact that
about three-quarters of the investigators using
the material are employing electron microscopy,
tissue culture, or biochemical technics.

Cooperation of the obstetrician and pathologist.
Besides the above mentioned technics of illus-
trating the laboratory's continuous interest in
the material, periodic reports and talks are
offered to the obstetricians. Short letters

describing each specimen are sent to each referring obstetrician, and in certain hospitals a
copy is sent to the record room for inclusion in
the mother's chart. Some reproductions of the
graphs of crown-rump length and gestational age
(Figure 1) have been used with attached advertise-
ments of the laboratory. If for health or
research reasons the parents should be contacted,
the personnel at the laboratory always approach
the patient through the obstetrician.

Specimens obtained from the operating room or
any fetal material are the responsibility of the
pathologist to examine. We are able in most
cases to remove material directly to the laboratory; however, in each situation a working
agreement with the pathologist is necessary.

Examination of the specimens. Historical information identifying the patient, referring doctor,
onset of last normal menstrual period and time of
passage are recorded; in most cases more detailed
information is not obtained unless volunteered by
the obstetrician or indicated by examination of
the specimen.

All specimens were examined by a physician and
the technics for measuring embryos and fetuses
have been previously described.[8,9,10] Crown-rump
and foot length are measured and in non-macerated
specimens, body and organ weights are recorded.
Well preserved specimens that fall within
Streeter's Horizons [11-14] (less than 34 mm. in
crown-rump length or about 54 gestational days)
are classified as embryos and for the most part
are used to enlarge our collection of serial
sections. We usually do obtain blood specimens
from them before fixation. Fetuses up to about
500 gm. of body weight are usually classified by
the referring obstetrician as a previable surgical type specimen. If the body weight is over
500 gm., permission for disposal by cremation and

burial permits are obtained.

A dissecting microscope is essential for removal of smaller organs in fetuses below 100 mm. in crown-rump length. Because of the very high water content of small fetuses and embryos, their shape and volume are maintained by carrying out the dissection in sterile Hanks solution. As many investigators receiving the material are using tissue culture technics, sterile instruments are used during the first part of the dissection.

The important judgment regarding the state of preservation or maceration requires a moderate amount of experience. If the heart is beating or from gross inspection the material is expected to have prophase mitotic figures, it is classified as excellent (grade I). If the material is suitable for gross anatomic examination without discoloration, distortion of the extremities, or collapse of the body cavities, it is classified as grade II. Other specimens are classified as macerated (grade III).

In the case of specimens obtained after curettage, the majority of time a foot can be identified and measured. From the foot length we convert to crown-rump length or weight (Figures 2 and 3) and from crown-rump length to gestational age.[10] As there are no useful organ weight standards with confidence levels for fetuses below 500 gm. of body weight, it was necessary to develop some from our own material.[15]

The determination of sex is done by one or more methods: 1) examination of external and internal organs, 2) direct aceto-orcein staining of amniotic nuclei and 3) karyotype, (infrequently). By the 60 mm. crown-rump stage we expect to see some fusion of the labia minora-like folds of the male phallus. The dissecting microscope is required for this judgment in specimens under about

90 mm. crown-rump length.

Costs. The laboratory is maintained on approximately $17,000 per year. This includes the salary of one technician and one secretary along with some supplies and equipment. The director, who expends about 10% of his time, is salaried from the University and postdoctoral fellows, who contribute about 20% of their time, are salaried from a training grant in human embryology and teratology.

The above tabulation is considered to represent a bare minimum; in other settings and with more sophisticated epidemiology the cost would be far greater.

IV TEACHING

The objectives of the collection have been in the major part directed toward education and research, a logical expectation in view of the unit's location in a university setting. The educational level reached extends from seventh and eighth graders to the mature scientific investigator. The high school groups benefit by the loan of human fetal specimens to their science teachers and in some cases by a tour of the laboratory collection. The mature investigators need information primarily on staging and description of the fetal material which they are using for their own studies. The main educational benefits have been for medical students and postdoctoral fellows. The medical students see many gross specimens. Also, personnel from the laboratory actively participate in teaching the medical embryology course. One of the main teaching materials in the human embryology course consists of student carousels composed of selected serial sections from a 9 mm. human embryo from the laboratory collection.

The postdoctoral fellows participate in the collection and description of the fresh material and in this way obtain a first-hand knowledge of early fetal pathology as well as human embryology. These persons are usually pediatricians who will use their embryology training in future academic careers in teratology.

V RESEARCH AND UTILIZATION

The number of specimens received per year has gradually increased from approximately 100 to 250 (Figure 4). The percentage of specimens from therapeutic abortion has increased from 12 to around 29; this upswing is related to increased public education about therapeutic abortion as well as a broadening of the medical criteria used by the local hospital committees on abortion.

Number and type of investigators supplied. The availability of fresh human fetal and embryonic material appears to have stimulated investigators to examine human material. Over 90 separate investigators have utilized the laboratory's material. Although the majority were from the Seattle area, eight were from other universities. The type of research technic used by these investigators can be roughly broken down into four categories: gross and light microscopic, 26%; electron microscopic, 18%; tissue culture, 24%; and biochemical, 32%.

The number of investigators using material varied according to the state of its preservation. After hysterotomy for therapeutic abortion, 84% of the specimens were distributed to five or more investigators with an average of 12 recipients. From therapeutic abortion by curettage, 65% of the specimens were used by five or more investigators with an average of eight. The fresh spontaneous specimens (grade I) were used by five or more investigators 69% of the time with an average of nine individuals. Only 20% of the grade II and 2% of grade III specimens could be utilized by five or more investigators.

Serial sectioned specimens. Our collection of serially sectioned human embryos number eighteen, of which one-half are of high quality. This loan collection has been used by a number of investigators for detailed studies and models of normal embryonic morphology. It may be of interest that over one-half of these early embryos were picked up during the night or weekends.

VI THE COLLECTION AND MONITORING

Advantages and an example. If an epidemic of malformations in the newborn should be accompanied by a rate increase in early abortions, a lead period of time amounting to six or seven months might be a very decided advantage as a warning. As an unexpected example from our own collection,[16] we noted a definite increase in therapeutic abortions for maternal rubella during the spring of 1965. This observation led to increased monitoring along with a research protocol for detection and study of the peak of rubella infected newborns when they reached birth six months later (Figure 5).

There is evidence that the malformation rate in therapeutic or spontaneous abortuses is higher than in the newborn.[1-7,17,18] It is reasonable then to suppose that this higher rate would be a more sensitive index to variations.

A third advantage to monitoring of abortuses is the ability to promptly obtain a history from the mother. It is possible, for instance, to interview the mother of an abortus with anencephaly within only a few weeks of the critical embryonic event. In the case of studies from the newborn, a period of seven or eight months separates the environmental events from the time of interview.

Problems. We have had the dilemma of choosing between a continued intake of sufficient numbers of specimens or more control over the completeness of the information about specimens. If the obstetrician or his nurse are asked or required to furnish too much information (and their time), they soon find excuses for not sending specimens. The invasion of their patient's privacy is often given as a legitimate reason for lack of cooperation.

The degree of post-mortem change in specimens has been a real problem in analysis of malformations. The pathologist's general lack of interest in products of conception may be due to the poor preservation of the tissues. Severely macerated specimens may exhibit absence of digits or portions of the skull which can be confused with adactyly or anencephaly.

The most difficult problem consists of ignorance about the size of the sample. How can we determine total sample size when we lack data on the number of ovulated ova which are subsequently fertilized, implanted, or implanted but aborted before the first missed menstrual period. In addition, the completeness of intake is an unknown variable. Our overall collection includes less than one-third of the expected specimens based on the number of live births. Even with the best hospital cooperation (a prepaid group who are interested in prevention), our abortion specimen rate is still only about 6% of the live newborns.

Other uncontrolled variables. The interest of the patient and doctor in the products of conception varies widely. A woman with several consecutive miscarriages is naturally more interested in what's going on; this increases our intake of specimens from habitual abortors. University Hospital personnel have a tendency to be less interested in sending specimens; the multiple non-routine requests weigh heavily on the work load of these university-based persons. The newborn with severe or rare malformation is selected by the obstetrician for referral; this causes an abnormally high incidence of malformations in the older segment of our intake. The obstetrical residents play an important role in our procurement of specimens and this may cause a lull in receipt during July when these physicians are coming onto new services. The day of the week and holidays also may have an effect on the rate of intake.

Research without hypotheses. Probably one of the most painful problems of monitoring a population is the lack of a specific testable hypothesis. This is all too evident to the more epidemiologic-oriented individuals. As an example, it should be pointed out that in the early phase of the thalidomide disaster when the mothers of phocomelic children were questioned about medication intake, the relationship of the defects to thalidomide was missed.[19] Later when a specific hypothesis about thalidomide was made, it was proven to be correct from repeat interviews of the same mothers.

VII SUMMARY

The methods used for establishing, maintaining and utilizing a collection of human embryonic and fetal specimens are discussed in detail. The objectives of the collection which were teaching, research and monitoring are evaluated.

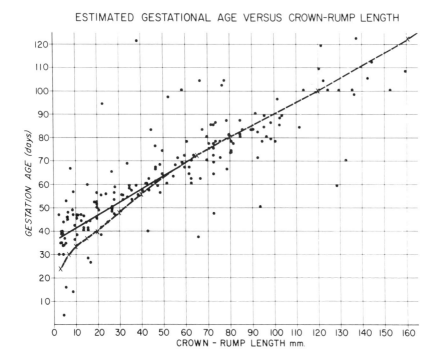

Figure 1. Gestational days in age plotted against crown-rump length. Data from therapeutic abortuses. The interrupted line below 40 mm. crown-rump is that of Streeter.[14] The approximation of our mean is the solid line. This material is much more fully treated by Iffey et al.[10]

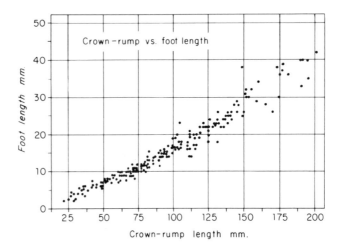

<u>Figure 2</u>. Foot length plotted against crown-rump length. From Shepard.[8] Courtesy W. B. Saunders Co., Philadelphia.

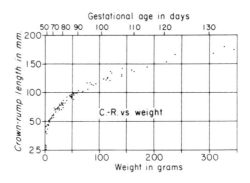

<u>Figure 3</u>. Crown-rump length plotted against weight. From Shepard.[8] Courtesy W. B. Saunders Co., Philadelphia.

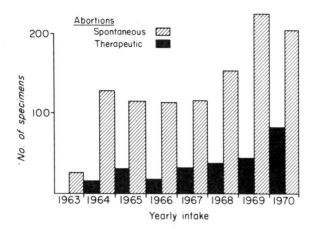

<u>Figure 4</u>. Yearly intake of therapeutic and spontaneous abortions. The years 1963 and 1970 are incomplete.

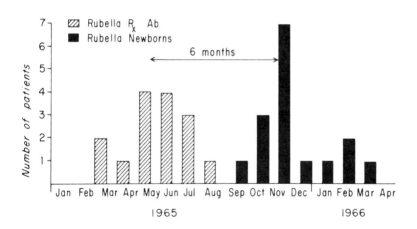

<u>Figure 5</u>. Rubella therapeutic abortion peak in the spring was a forewarning of an epidemic of the rubella syndrome in the newborn six months later. (From Shepard and Hollingsworth.[16] Courtesy Amer. Acad. of Pediatrics.)

COLLECTION OF HUMAN EMBRYOS AND FETUSES

A Centralized Laboratory for Collection
of Human Embryos and Fetuses: Seven Years Experience: II. Classification and Tabulation of
Conceptual Wastage with Observations on Type of
Malformation, Sex Ratio and Chromosome Studies.[1]

Thomas Nelson[2]
Godfrey P. Oakley, Jr.[3]
Thomas H. Shepard

1. Supported by grants from the National
    Institutes of Health (HD00836,
    5-T01-HD-00180 and DE02918).

2. Postdoctoral Research Trainee
    supported by grant 5-T01-HE0180
    from the National Institutes of
    Health.

3. Supported by Department of Health
    Education and Welfare, Public
    Health Services and Mental Health
    Administration Center for Disease
    Control.

OUTLINE

I INTRODUCTION

There have been relatively few collections of spontaneously aborted human material. Descriptions of these collections have been difficult to compare because of differences in methods of gestational age assignment and lack of uniform morphological classifications. As more of these collections are being started, it has become apparent that the types of material collected are not always strictly comparable.

In this paper we shall demonstrate some of the problems that occur in trying to obtain and describe a representative sample of human abortuses. We also hope to show that the difficulty in comparing various series can be reduced by using accurate gestational dating and by adopting a simple but consistant morphological classification. Sample abortus populations are often far from uniformly representative of the population of all human abortuses and thus it is imperative to have some idea of the selective biases that may occur in any collection.

The material analyzed in this paper was derived from our collection of 1365 products of conception obtained over a seven year period. After excluding induced abortions, 13 ectopic pregnancies and twins and triplets, 1038 specimens remain which were suitable for classification.

The material has been divided into two large groups for classification and analysis because one hospital, Hospital A, submitted a more complete sample of conceptual wastage from its patient population. This sample, therefore, gives a more accurate picture of the biology of fetal and embryonic wastage. Hospital A, a pre-payment plan group, submitted abortuses in the last year at a rate of 60 per 1000 live births; during the last four years, it submitted 272 specimens. The other hospitals donated 766 abortuses over the last seven years.

II CLASSIFICATION AND TABULATION

Description of classification. The general classification adopted below is closely analogous to that proposed by Fujikura et al.,[3] in 1966. This classification allows the material to be separated into useful groups which have certain characteristics in common, without relying on morphologic alterations which may turn out to be of questionable significance.

Group I: Incomplete specimens. Specimens consisting of villi or decidua containing trophoblastic cells. Such material is commonly obtained from curetting after an incomplete abortion.

Group II: Ruptured chorionic sacs without embryos.
A) Chorionic sacs with umbilical cord stump.
B) Chorionic sacs without evidence of a cord.

Group III: Intact chorionic sacs without embryos.

Group IV: A large group which included all specimens which had an embryo or fetus or a recognizable fragment of the embryo or fetus. This group was further divided into four subgroups.
A) Normal embryos or fetuses.
B) Embryonic growth retardation which includes specimens previously described as nodular and cylindrical. (These small embryos are so grossly deformed that they have few recognizable morphologic features).

Stunted embryos are included in this
group.
C) Embryos and fetuses with localized anomalies or recognizable
syndromes. This subgroup would
contain embryos with neural tube
defects, multiple recognizable
malformations and syndromes such as
Turner's syndrome.
D) Specimens of embryonic or fetal
tissue which were too fragmented or
too autolysed to make a determination as to the normality or
abnormality of the conceptus.

Specimens were assigned a gestational age by
measuring the crown-rump length (or foot-length
in damaged fetuses) or by morphologic features
consistant with Streeter's horizons.

All growth-retarded embryos (IVB) and ruptured
or intact sac were arbitrarily assigned to the
youngest age group since death had probably
occurred in this period. Such specimens are frequently retained in utero for considerable
periods.

Our morphological groups are identical with
Fujikura's but for these exceptions: All group I
material was assigned an unknown age group.
Many of the descriptions of our empty sacs did
not mention the presence or absence of a cord.
All cases without mention of a cord are placed in
group IIB, though a few may have indeed had cords.
Unless the description clearly indicated that a
chorionic sac was ruptured, the specimen was
assigned to group III along with the adequately-
described, intact sacs. The completeness of
examination of the specimens varied. A specimen
was classified normal if there was no neural
tube defect, cleft palate, digital defect nor
external features suggesting a known disease or

syndrome. If an internal malformation was found in an externally normal fetus, it was classified as abnormal. Fetuses were placed in a non-classified group if their description made no statement about their morphology. Fujikura et al.,[3] also placed their stunted embryos in the IVA category rather than in IVB.

Classification of material by age group. Table I contrasts the age distribution of our material as percentages of the two hospital subgroups. We emphasize this contrast to illustrate the marked effect that selection may have on the distribution of types of conceptuses. The two subgroups appear to be similar in some age categories but quite different in others. Conceptuses from the embryonic period constitute 48.9% of the material from Hospital A as compared to 28.4% from the other contributing hospitals. Some of the incomplete decidual casts with villus fragments classified under unknown age may well represent remains of embryonic aberrations, and if this group were added, the percentage of embryonic abortuses would be even higher in the Hospital A series. Conversely, in the age period of 92-126 days a wide discrepancy between the two groups exists in that the group A collection contained only 8.4% as compared to 26.8% for material from other hospitals. The different distribution of material by gestational age between our groups is likely the result of methods used by the various hospitals to select the material that they donated to our laboratory rather than some inherent biological difference among the patients.

Morphological classification by age. Table 2 shows the morphologic distribution by age for our collection. Chorionic sacs without embryos (II plus III) comprise 48.8% of our material from the embryonic period for Hospital A compared to 27.5%

from the other hospitals. In addition to these differences, 14% of the specimens from Hospital A were decidual material with villi compared with 4.6% of the material from our other hospitals. These discrepancies again suggest some selective bias toward normal embryos by personnel in the other hospitals.

Comparison of morphological distribution of this collection with other previously described series. Most of the previous classifications of spontaneously aborted conceptuses had been patterned after Mall and Meyer,[1] and Hertig.[2] Fujikura et al.,[3] further modified Hertig's classification to the general form which was adopted in this present report. Table 3 has been constructed using Fujikura's scheme to allow comparison where possible with other series. Fujikura et al., classify their material by menstrual age rather than by size or stage. This does indeed serve to emphasize the fact that many products of conception are retained for long periods after death, but it does not allow an accurate appraisal of the stage at which the material dies. The developmental period at the time of death seems to us to contribute potentially the most toward analysis of the various etiologies.

Despite this difference in approach, there are no radical differences between our material (Hospital A) and that of Fujikura. Furthermore, our percentage of intact empty sacs agrees reasonably well with that of others (Fujikura,[3] Stratford,[7] Singh and Carr,[4] Mikamo,[6] MacMahon[20]). The overall percentage of normal fetuses fits with those reported in other series (Fujikura,[3] Stratford,[7] MacMahon[20]) and likewise our percentage of localized abnormalities agree closely with the series of Mall and Meyer.[1] Both Poland[5] and Stratford[7] demonstrated by routinely autopsying all fetuses that the percentage of localized anomalies may be increased considerably over what had previously been reported. The discrepancy between our percentage of localized abnormalities and these investigators is probably explained in part by the strong selective forces which altered their distribution to such a great extent that no ruptured sacs and very few empty intact sacs were observed.

III LACK OF SEASONAL TRENDS

The last menstrual period was known for approximately 75% of the abortions received over the last three years. Three hundred and four spontaneous abortions less than 175 mm. crown-rump length were conceived between July 1967 and June 1970. There was no seasonal trend noted, but a gradual increase in the number of specimens was found. No significant seasonal trend was noted when the last 18 months of data was reviewed from Hospital A.

IV INCIDENCE AND TYPE OF LOCALIZED MALFORMATION

Eighty-seven fetuses and embryos (8.4%) of the total 1,038 specimens reviewed in our laboratory had localized abnormalities which are detailed in Table 4. Each specimen is represented only once in the Table. Those with multiple malformations were recorded as a syndrome or by the most serious defect. All observations were made independently of chromosomal analysis.

The percentage of embryos and fetuses with localized malformations among reported fetal wastage series varies (IVC in Table 3). Fujikura et al.,[3] reported 1.8%, MacMahon et al.,[20] reported 2.0%, while Stratford[7] recently reported 27.1%. Our 8.2% is near the 7.5% found in Mall and Meyer's[1] report. The comparisons of these percentages among various series is of little value because much of the variation observed is a function of what segment of the total embryonic and fetal wastage is presented to the various investigators for review. A conclusion, however, seems justified: the percentage of embryos and fetuses with localized malformations among spontaneous abortions is higher than that found in the newborn.

In our series, as in that of Mall and Meyer,[1] the most frequent localized anomalies are neural tube defects. Anencephaly, spina bifida and exencephaly occurred in 35 per 1000 of Mall and Meyer's[1] specimens and 36 per 1000 of our specimens. Our series contain more older fetuses with neural tube defects because Dr. Ronald Lemire has actively solicited these specimens from the community.

The incidence of neural tube defects has been shown to vary among certain geographic and ethnic newborn populations.[21] Perhaps the absolute number of conceptuses with neural tube defects is a constant, but varying degrees of fetal wastage among populations may produce the observed differences in newborn incidence. This problem can only be solved by quantitating the incidence of these malformations over the entire gestational period. In comparison with Mall and Meyer[1] our series is deficient in the number of cases of cyclopia and conjoined twins. Our series, on the other hand, contained a large number of clinical Turner's syndrome (7.7 per 1000 specimens) and exstrophy of the cloaca (4.8 per 1000 specimens). Another seven cases of XO syndrome not included in Table 4 were identified chromosomally. Further investigations of such regional differences in incidence rates of specific defects may shed light on the etiology of these diseases.

V TWINS AND TRIPLETS

We received 47 products of twin conceptions
(21 pairs, five single members). The 11 (32%)
that were abnormal included five acardiac monsters, one female with Turner's phenotype and
chromosomal confirmation, one pair of thoracopa-
gus conjoined twins, one fetus with congenital
glaucoma and polydactly and two amorphous embryos.
The normal members of a set of triplets were
examined.

VI SEX RATIOS

No significant differences in sex ratio were
noted in our relatively small number of specimens
(Table 5). A slightly significant predominance
of males in the 51 to 150 mm. group was found
after the first four years of collecting. This
was not apparent after subsequent specimens were
added; we attribute this to more experience on
our part and especially to the use of a
dissecting microscope for examination of the external and internal genitalia. The very high
male to female ratio found in older studies has
gradually dropped as more accurate observation
has been used.[22]
The results of sex ratio studies in early
abortuses can be easily modified by subtle errors
in technic. Mikamo[23] has accurately described
and pictured the gross changes in the external
and internal genitalia of early human fetuses and
the use of his standards is recommended. When
the nuclear sex chromatin method is used before
sexual differentiation, it is possible to obtain
a falsely high number of females because, in
general, a preparation without obvious nuclear
bodies is more liable to be judged as not read-
able thus discarding more borderline males

than females. In the embryonic period, as we
point out below, there is a serious problem of
excluding contamination of cultures with maternal
cells from the placenta. These two errors would
add to the proportion of females in the early
material. A third factor is the incidence of XO
abortuses which could be classified as males by
the nuclear chromatin method. Carr[24] has
reported this to be about 5% of spontaneous early
abortuses. In summary, the sex ratio of early
abortus material should be based on karyotyped
cultures obtained with special care from the
embryo.

VII CHROMOSOMES FROM THE ABORTUSES

Chromosomes from the abortuses. Over roughly a
three year period, 124 cell cultures from abortuses were initiated and of these 71 (57%)
developed sufficient growth for chromosome analysis. (The karyotype analyses were performed
under the supervision of Dr. Stanley Gartler and
Mrs. Jean Bryant, Departments of Medicine and
Genetics, University of Washington.) Eighteen
(25%) of the karyotypes were abnormal. The
chromosomes from conceptuses estimated to be 56
days or less had a higher incidence of abnormality (45%) than larger specimens (14%).

Oral contraceptives and karyotype. The mothers
of 33 karyotyped abortuses were interviewed regarding use of oral contraceptives. In eight
instances the mothers had been using oral contraceptives within six months of conceiving the
abortus. Four of these eight were abnormal
including one triploid, two XO's, and one deletion of the short arm of an E chromosome.
These findings did not significantly differ from
the results from abortuses of 25 women who had
not taken oral contraception within six months of

conceiving. In this group of 25, there were 11 abnormal, three triploids, four XO's, three trisomes (F,B and 18) and one D monosomy. These results differ from those reported by Carr[24] who found an increase in polyploidy in abortuses obtained within six months of oral contraception.

The sex ratio of all fetuses successfully cultured was weighted heavily toward the females with 39 females to 19 males (excluding polyploidys and XO's). We believe this difference is artifactual depending on the source of the culture. Of 15 cultures grown from placentas, 14 were female while of 36 cultures grown from embryonic material only 23 were female.

Closing comments. As we have reviewed our own data and the published work of others, we have been made aware of many collection problems associated with the establishment and maintenance of a collection such as ours and of the difficulties in the interpretation of the data collected. We have also been reminded of the quantity of pathology in the spontaneous abortions that can be defined by the careful observations and chromosomal analysis. We agree with Dr. David H. Carr:[24]

"The introduction of abortion registries accompanied by detailed pregnancy histories could contribute greatly to our understanding of the mechanisms underlying congenital defects. The great majority of defective offspring are spontaneously aborted and the period of recall of events is much shorter than for pregnancies going to term. This valuable aborted material is literally down the drain, and we need to correct this omission if environmental disasters or benefits in relation to pregnancy are to be detected."

VIII SUMMARY

A retrospective classification of our material by the method of Fujikura et al.,[3] has allowed comparison with previously reported series. Types of malformations in our collection have been discussed and results of our chromosomal analysis have been presented. The sex ratio in our series does not show a significant difference. Review of our spontaneous abortuses has shown that there are differences between the collection we have obtained from Hospital A and that obtained from other hospitals. We believe these differences to be brought about by methods of sample selection. Similar selective biases contribute to difficulty in comparing different reported series.

ACKNOWLEDGEMENTS

We gratefully acknowledge Dr. Ralph Hollingsworth who helped in the collection and description of specimens. The laboratory advisory committee which was so helpful in the initial stages was composed of Drs. Charles Hunter, Arno Motulsky, Richard Blandau and Donald McIntyre. We appreciate the help of a large number of obstetricians and in particular personnel from the following hospitals: Group Health Hospital, Swedish Hospital Medical Center, University of Washington Hospital and King County-Harborview Hospital. Mrs. Dian Lowinger and Mrs. Linda Quan Knight, two University of Washington medical students, interviewed the parents in the chromosome studies.

REFERENCES

1. Mall, F. P., Meyer, A.W.: Studies on abortuses: a survey of pathological ova in the Carnegie embryological collection. Contr. Embryol. 12:5-364, 1921.

2. Hertig, A., Sheldon, W.H.: Minimal criteria required to prove prima facie case of traumatic abortion: an analysis of 1,000 spontaneous abortions. Annals of Surgery 117: 596-606, 1943.

3. Fujikura, T., Froehlich, L.A., Driscoll, S.G.: A simplified anatomic classification of abortions. Amer.J.Obst.& Gyn. 95: 902-905, 1966.

4. Singh, R.P., Carr, D.H.: Anatomic findings in human abortions of known chromosomal constitution. Obstet. Gynec. 29:806-818, 1967.

5. Poland, B.J.: Study of developmental anomalies in the spontaneously aborted fetus. Amer.J.Obst.& Gyn.105:501-505, 1968.

6. Mikamo, K.: Anatomic and chromosomal anomalies in spontaneous abortion. Am.J.Obst.& Gyn. 106:243-254, 1970.

7. Stratford, B.F.: Abnormalities of early human development. Amer.J.Obst.& Gyn. 107: 1223-1232, 1970.

8. Shepard, T.H.: In Endocrine and Genetic diseases of Children, edited by L.I.Gardner, Philadelphia, W.B.Saunders Co., pp.1-6,1969.

9. Shepard, T.H.: Prenatal Factors, Endocrine and Metabolic Disorders in Children. Edited by V.C.Kelley. In press, New York, Paul B. Hoeber & Co.

10. Iffy, L., Shepard, T.H., Jakobovits, A. et al.: The rate of growth in young human embryos of Streeter's horizons XIII to XXIII. Acta. Anat. 66:178-186, 1967.

11. Streeter, G.L.: Developmental horizons in human embryos. Description of age groups XI, 13-20 somites and age group XII, 21-19 somites. Contr. Embryol. 30:211-145, 1942.

12. Streeter, G.L.: Developmental horizons in human embryos. Description of age groups XIII, embryos about 4 or 5 millimeters long and age group XIV, period of indentation of the lens vesicle. Contr. Embryol. 31:27-63, 1945.

13. Streeter, G.L.: Developmental horizons in human embryos. Description of age groups XV, XVI, XVIII, being the third of a survey of the Carnegie Collection. Contr. Embryol. 32:133-203, 1948.

14. Streeter, G.L.: Developmental horizons in known embryos. Description of age groups XIX, XX, XXI, XXII and XXIII, being the fifth issue of a survey of the Carnegie Collection. Contr. Embryol. 34:165-196, 1951.

15. Tanimura, T., Nelson, T., Hollingsworth, R.R. et al.: Weight standards for organs from early fetuses. Submitted for publication, 1970.

16. Shepard, T.H., Hollingsworth, R.R.: Teratologic monitoring through embryo and fetus collecting. Letter to editor. Pediat. 42: 713-714, 1968.

17. Nishimura, H., Takano, K., Tanimura, T. et al.: High incidence of several malformations in early human embryos as compared with infants. Biol. Neonat. 10:93-107, 1966.

18. Nishimura, H., Takano, K., Tanimura, T. et al.: Normal and abnormal development of human embryos: first report of the analysis of 1,213 intact embryos. Teratology 1:281-290, 1968.

19. Speirs, A.L.: Thalidomide and congenital

abnormalities. Lancet 1:303-305, 1962.
20. MacMahon, B., Hertig, A., Ingalls, T.: Association between maternal age and pathologic diagnosis in abortion: Obst. & Gynec. 4:477-483, 1954.
21. Naggan, L., MacMahon, B.: Ethnic difference in the prevalence of anencephaly and spina bifida in Boston, Massachusetts. New Eng. J. Med. 277:119-123, 1967.
22. Tietze, C.: A note on the sex ratio of abortions. Human Biol. 20:156-160, 1948.
23. Mikamo, K.: Prenatal sex ratio in man: observations contradictory to prevailing concepts. Obst. & Gynec. 34:710-716, 1969.
24. Carr, D.H.: Chromosome studies in selected spontaneous abortions; 1. Conception after oral contraceptives. Canad. Med. Ass. J. 103:343-348, 1970.

Table 1

COMPARATIVE DISTRIBUTION OF SPONTANEOUS ABORTIONS
ACCORDING TO GESTATIONAL AGE

Gestational Age Range in Days (Weeks)	Hospital A	Our Other Hospitals
15-56 (2-8)	133 (48.9)*	218 (28.4)*
57-91 (9-13)	39 (14.3)	147 (19.2)
92-126 (14-18)	23 (8.4)	205 (26.8)
Above 126 (>19)	38 (14.0)	151 (19.7)
Unknown	39 (14.3)	45 (5.9)
All Ages	272 (100)	766 (100)

* Percentages of each group

Table 2

CLASSIFICATION AND TABULATION OF SPONTANEOUS ABORTIONS OBTAINED FROM HOSPITAL "A" AND OUR OTHER HOSPITALS

Gestational Age Range in Days (Weeks)	Hospital	Incomplete Specimen	Ruptured Sacs Without Embryos		Intact Sacs Without Embryos	Embryos or Fetus Present				Not Classified	Total Reported
			No Cord			Normal	Embryonic Growth Retardation	Localized Abnormality	Cannot Determine Normal		
		I	Cord II A	II B	III	IV A	IV B	IV C	IV D		
15-56 (2-8)	A	0 (0)	16.5 (22)*	15.8 (21)*	16.5 (22)*	18.0 (24)*	14.3 (19)*	1.5 (2)*	17.3 (23)*		100 (%) (133)*
	Others	0 (0)	4.1 (9)	11.0 (24)	12.4 (27)	34.9 (76)	10.1 (22)	4.6 (10)	22.0 (48)	0.9 (2)*	100 (218)
57-91 (9-13)	A					59.0 (23)		15.4 (6)	25.6 (10)		100 (39)
	Others					79.6 (117)		6.8 (10)	13.6 (20)		100 (147)
92-126 (14-18)	A					82.6 (19)		8.7 (2)	8.7 (2)		100 (23)
	Others					84.9 (174)		5.4 (11)	6.8 (14)	2.9 (6)	100 (205)
> 126 (< 19)	A					57.9 (22)		23.7 (9)	18.4 (7)		100 (38)
	Others					66.9 (101)		23.8 (36)	2.6 (4)	6.6 (10)	100 (151)
Unknown	A	97.4 (38)							2.6 (1)		100 (39)
	Others	77.8 (35)				2.2 (1)				20.0 (9)	100 (45)
Total of all Ages	A	14.0 (38)	8.1 (22)	7.7 (21)	8.1 (22)	32.3 (88)	7.0 (19)	7.0 (19)	15.8 (43)		100 (272)
	Others	4.6 (35)	1.2 (9)	3.1 (24)	3.5 (27)	61.2 (469)	2.9 (22)	8.7 (67)	11.2 (86)	3.5 (27)	100 (766)

*Number of Specimens in Each Group

Table 3

RECLASSIFICATION OF OTHER REPORTED SERIES OF EMBRYONIC AND FETAL WASTAGE AND COMPARISON WITH OUR COLLECTION

Hospital	Incomplete Specimens I	Ruptured Sacs Without Embryos — Cord II A	Ruptured Sacs Without Embryos — No Cord II B	Intact Sacs Without Embryos III	Embryos or Fetus Present — Normal IV A	Embryos or Fetus Present — Embryonic Growth Retardation IV B	Embryos or Fetus Present — Localized Abnormality IV C	Embryos or Fetus Present — Cannot Determine Normal IV D	Not Classified	Total Reported (%)
Hospital A	14.8 (40)*	8.1 (22)*	7.7 (21)*	8.1 (22)*	32.5 (88)*	7.0 (19)*	7.0 (19)*	14.8 (40)*		100 (271)*
Our Other Hospital	3.9 (30)	1.2 (9)	3.1 (24)	3.5 (27)	61.2 (469)	3.0 (23)	8.7 (67)	11.7 (90)	3.5 (27)*	100 (766)
Mall and Meyer[1]	3.6 (36)	←—— 9.2 (92) ——→			56.7 (567)	18.2 (182)	7.5 (75)	4.8 (48)		100 (1000)
MacMahon et al.[23]	2.3 (28)	←—— 32.6 (398) ——→		10.9 (133)	39.3 (480)	12.9 (157)	2.0 (24)	0 (0)		100 (1220)
Fujikura et al.[3]	22.0 (72)	4.0 (13)	23.5 (77)	5.5 (18)	35.8+ (117)	4.0 (13)	1.8 (6)	3.4 (11)		100 (327)
Poland[5]	0 (0)	0 (0)	0 (0)	2.4 (3)	56.8 (71)	16.0 (20)	24.8 (31)	0 (0)		100 (125)
Singh and Carr[4]	?	←—— 17.8 (69) ——→		12.9 (50)	?	?	?	?	69.3 (278)	100 (387)
Mikamo[6]	?	?	?	9.4 (30)	66.7 (212)	?	12.3 (39)	?		100 (318)
Stratford[7]	7.1 (15)	0	0	7.6 (16)	37.6 (76)	20.5 (43)	27.1 (57)	0		100 (210)

* Number of specimens in each group
+ Stunted embryos were included in this group

62

Table 4

EMBRYOS AND FETUSES WITH LOCALIZED ABNORMALITIES BY GESTATIONAL AGE

Type of Abnormality	15-56 Days (2-8 Weeks)	57-91 Days (9-13 Weeks)	92-126 Days (14-18 Weeks)	>126 Days (>19 Weeks)	Total
Chromosomal Syndromes					
Turner's	0	0	5	3	8
Trisomy 18	0	0	0	2	2
Central Nervous System					
Anencaphaly	7	3	0	21	31
Spina bifida	4	0	1	1	6
Hydrocephalus	0	1	0	3	4
Gastrointestinal System					
Cleft lip +/- palate	1	3	1	0	5
Cleft palate	0	2	0	0	2
Exstrophy of cloaca	0	1	2	2	5
Omphalocele	0	0	1	0	1
Urogenital System	0	4	0	4	8
Cardiovascular System					
Atrial septal defect	0	0	0	1	1
Ventricular septal defect	0	1	0	0	1
Musculoskeletal System					
Achondroplasia	0	0	0	2	2
Congenital amputation	0	0	0	2	2
Polydactyly	0	1	2	0	3
Syndactyly	0	0	1	0	1
Sirenomelia	0	0	0	2	2
Other					
Sacrococcygeal teratoma	0	0	0	1	1
Total Anomalies	12 (3.4%)	16 (8.6%)	13 (5.7%)	44 (23.3%)	85 (8.2%)
Total Specimens	351	186	228	189	1,038*

*Includes 84 specimens with unknown gestational age.

Table 5

SEX RATIOS FROM SPONTANEOUS AND THERAPEUTIC
ABORTIONS

Length Crown-Rump MM	Spontaneous		Therapeutic	
	Male	Female	Male	Female
0-50	37	44	20	26
51-100	74	74	36	23
101-150	110	89	19	12
151 and over	128	154	11	8
	349	361	86	69

MONITORING OF HUMAN EMBRYONIC AND FETAL WASTAGE[*]

James R. Miller
Betty J. Poland[**]

The question of "Why Monitor?" has been
answered by Dr. Murphy in the first paper of this
Symposium, but it undoubtedly will be raised
again a number of times. There might be a
tendency in the minds of some people to group the
type of problem we are discussing here with the
general question of screening programmes for the
early detection of disease states. I mention
this because there has been recent discussion
about such projects and criticism has been made
that the cost-benefit ratios in some instances
are not adequate enough to justify their inclusion in general health service schemes. The
problem we are tackling, that of surveillance,
has a different goal. Rather than aim at early
detection for the purpose of initiating treatment
services, surveillance is concerned with early
detection for the purpose of being alert to the
presence of new teratogens or mutagens in the

---

[*]The original work referred to in this
presentation was made possible by a Grant from
the Medical Research Council of Canada, #MA-2740.
[**]Department of Obstetrics and Gynaecology,
University of British Columbia.

environment. Although this difference may be self-evident, it is one that must be stressed because the criteria for evaluating surveillance schemes will be quite different from those used to evaluate screening programs.

Newcombe[1] has recently set forth the following three criteria for efficient surveillance schemes designed for the detection of new teratogens:

1. a high degree of specificity in diagnosis and classification of anomalies;

2. early detection of anomalies; and

3. improved methods for the recording, rapid accumulation and communication of data on such anomalies.

It is obvious that Newcombe's criteria are put forth for schemes which will involve the use of data derived from the examination of live and stillborn infants. Despite the fact that such data are easy to come by because of the legal obligation associated with the recording of the birth of term or near term infants, it is our thesis that surveillance schemes should not be confined to observations made at this time but should be designed to detect evidence of new teratogens as early as possible through the inclusion in monitoring systems of aborted embryos and fetuses. It should be stressed that it is our assumption that such a programme using observations on embryos and fetuses is part of a larger one which includes data derived from live and stillbirths, neonatal deaths, etc.[2,3]

Since there are some obvious problems associated with the use of embryos and fetuses in a surveillance scheme, there may be some justifiable concern about the value of including them at all. In our opinion there are four principal reasons for their inclusion:

1. The events which we are so anxious to detect and study occur during the embryonic

and fetal periods of development.

2. Developmental anomalies occur in abortuses with approximately ten times the frequency with which they occur in term births, and there is no reason to suspect that the mechanisms for their production differs in the two groups.

3. The closing of the time gap between the initiating events of anomalous developmental processes and the time these processes are observed and recorded is an absolute essential of a good surveillance scheme (see Newcombe's criterion #2 above). The use of observations made at term means that in most instances a time lag of nine months or longer exists between the initiating event and the time of recording. The inclusion of abortuses would reduce this time lag significantly.

4. It is essential to minimize the maternal and physician memory bias associated with events occurring during early pregnancy. Anyone who has been associated with the collection of retrospective information is aware of the problems posed by the distortion of events and their timing which occur in the minds of informants with the passage of time. The use of embryos and fetuses reduces the time interval between the occurrence of any outstanding event which might be of etiological significance and the time at which "the alarm bell" of a monitoring system rings.

As an example of the rewards of narrowing the time between the initiating event and the observation, I should like to summarize a case from our own studies on prenatal developmental anomalies.

The 22 year old mother was Para I, Gravida II, and exhibited clinical evidence of rubella at 137 days (19 weeks) of pregnancy. This was confirmed by a rising titre of rubella antibodies during the seven days following the onset of the rash.

An abdominal hysterotomy was performed at 163 days. The fetus was a female measuring 157 mms. crown-rump length, which was appreciably smaller than was expected for a gestational age of 163 days, and there was suggestion of growth retardation. The fetus, developmentally, corresponded to a gestational age of 147 days and a developmental age of 120 days. There were no external anomalies, but internally there was a coarctation of the aorta, a subvalvular pulmonary stenosis and a ventricular septal defect. There is no way, from our present knowledge of the development of the heart, in which the rubella virus acting during the 15th to 16th week (the earliest time it was possible in view of the accurate documentation involved) could have produced these cardiac malformations. We believe that if the specimen had gone to term the heart defect would have been attributed incorrectly to the rubella episode, and indeed from the evidence available this opinion would have been justified.

It should be pointed out that even a rather sophisticated system of record linkage would not overcome the problems associated with accuracy of retrospective information retrieval on such a sequence of events, because most of the events with which we are concerned are the type that often do not get recorded in any formal records (e.g. hospital or laboratory records and physicians' notes) but are in the mother's or physicians' memory store which are notoriously poor sources for sound information retrieval.

Problems in the Use of Embryos and Fetuses

Any advocate of the use of embryos and fetuses in a surveillance programme must be prepared to face the challange of the many problems associated with the collection and examination of such material. A major problem centers around the question of determining precisely what the population of specimens under examination represents. Live and stillbirths represent biological events which are reportable by law. Therefore, the total number of individuals at risk is recorded relatively accurately in a routine fashion for most populations, even though the accuracy of the extimate of the true number of individuals with a specific defect will vary depending upon the methods of ascertainment used in a given surveillance programme. However, there are no legal obligations governing the reporting of products of conception prior to 20 - 24 weeks, and thus it is virtually impossible to determine with any reasonable degree of accuracy the total population at risk prior to these dates. Nishimura has made some gross estimates of some of these parameters based on his extensive studies of Japanese abortuses.[4]

Carr[5] has recently suggested that abortions should be notifiable events, and that the record should include data on anomalies and a record of abnormal events occurring during the pregnancy. Although we would agree completely with this idea it should be recognized that in view of the difficulties associated with the routine reporting of data relating to stillbirths it would appear to be a formidable task to institute an effective scheme for the routine reporting of abortuses. Even if such a routine reporting scheme were established which could be used for the collection of monitoring data it would still be impossible to collect all abortuses. Since under a postulated ideal system it would not be possible to obtain data on all specimens at risk, the question remains as to what specimens are more desirable, and what are the attendant biases associated with taking samples.

Therapeutic versus Spontaneous Abortuses

Samples of abortuses obtained by therapeutic intervention have several potential biases. Although there are a variety of techniques which can be used in abortion procedures, most of these result in some damage to the specimen. In particular techniques used in the early stages of pregnancy cause severe damage and hence specimens under three months would be under-represented in the total sample. Do all specimens have an equal probability of being damaged in this way, or are specimens with developmental anomalies more prone to damage or destruction? Regardless of the answer, certainly the fact that damage occurs in a high percentage of all cases would reduce the potential sample considerably. In personal conversation with Dr. Nishimura and members of his group in Kyoto it appears that only about 2% of the specimens obtained by them in their study of therapeutically aborted embryos and fetuses are intact specimens that are totally free of any damage.

The frequency of developmental anomalies observed in therapeutic abortuses will be less than that found in spontaneous abortuses. Table I compares the frequency of anomalous cases observed in our study amongst abortuses obtained in various ways. The general observation of a graded decrease in frequency of defects in spontaneous abortuses through to newborns has been commented on by Nishimura and his colleagues.[4,6] The question we should like to pose to statisticians is "From what baseline is it easier to detect significant changes or does it not matter as long as reliable baseline estimates are chosen?".

Not only will the frequency of anomalous specimens differ depending upon the type of abortuses used but also the types of anomalous events observed. While many of the anomalies observed in abortuses cover the same general spectrum observed in term infants there are a group of defects which are found exclusively in spontaneously aborted embryos. These are the specimens with growth disorganization. In our series of 223 abnormal specimens, 111 (or 50%) had such defects, and of these, 96 (43% of the total sample sample) were embryos (under 30 mms. crown-rump length).[2]

Another bias posed by the use of specimens obtained by therapeutic intervention revolves around the legal restrictions on this operation. In those communities where the abortion law is quite liberal all pregnant women would have access theoretically to the operation but not all women would take advantage of this opportunity. What are the characteristics of the group of women who do not utilize the service, and what is the relevance of these characteristics to the problem of surveillance? For instance, in Canada the abortion law, while quite restrictive, is interpreted with a fair degree of flexibility in many parts of the country. At the present time the population of women seeking this operation in British Columbia comprises overwhelmingly the single girl under 20 years and the older multiparous. In those communities where the risk of producing an abnormal infant constitutes grounds for abortion procedures, provision would have to be made for the elimination of such cases from any monitoring scheme, or if they were not eliminated there would have to be an awareness of the potential bias introduced by such cases if they were numerous.

In the case of spontaneous abortuses there are also obvious biases. Most early losses are missed, and no system of routine reporting is likely to correct this loss. This is not too

disturbing because it is generally recognized
that the frequency of developmental anomalies in
these specimens is probably close to 90%, and is
therefore a poor baseline from which to begin
looking for significant increases.

What women come into the hospital with threat-
ened abortion? Obviously a very large percentage
will comprise those who want to save their
pregnancy and those who because of excess hem-
orrhaging or other serious medical problems need
special hospital nursing care. These factors are
probably associated with a population of women
with certain biological characteristics. Although we do not believe that there is any
identifiable factor in our studies that would
produce a major bias in a surveillance programme
the possibility of potential biases stemming from
these characteristics must be considered. It
should also be emphasized that these biases may
change with time as laws or medical practice
change, or as the structure of society, i.e. the
socio-economic class from which the sample
derives, changes.

Almost all spontaneous abortuses have some
degree of maceration because only a few known
causes of spontaneous abortion (e.g. incompetent
cervix) will yield a fresh specimen. In any
monitoring programme there must be provision for
careful evaluation of distinguishing between
spontaneous developmental errors and post-mortem
changes. In general, maceration produces distortion and makes dissection difficult. Therefore, for complete study of such specimens
fixation is necessary. If a specimen has a defect, such as ventricular septal defect, the
distortion produced by maceration will not change
this. In general, while it must be acknowledged
that the maceration associated with almost all
spontaneous abortuses makes for problems, if care

is excercised we believe that distortion induced
by this reason can be distinguished from true
anomalous development in the vast majority of
cases.

When all factors are considered it is our
personal opinion that the collection of therapeutic abortuses represents a great deal of
effort for relatively small returns, and that for
purposes of a surveillance programme spontaneous
abortuses are far more useful.

Suggested Design of a Surveillance Scheme

We have been asked to comment on the costs
associated with the inclusion of abortuses in a
surveillance programme. Although we have considered seriously the matter for a long time we
are unable to come up with meaningful figures.
Our own programme is designed as a research
project with goals which are quite different from
those of monitoring schemes. Perhaps it is more
relevant to discuss some elements which we think
are important in the use of abortuses in a surveillance programme:

1. Collecting specimens and obtaining pregnancy data. In our opinion the specimens should
be collected and delivered daily to a pathology
laboratory for routine processing. At the same
time each specimen is collected, information on
the pregnancy should be obtained. This may seem
an unnecessary aspect of a scheme designed for
monitoring where speed is an important component.
However, in any surveillance scheme the critical
aspect is not the sounding of "the alarm bell"
but the initiation of follow up procedures once
the warning is given. Such follow up procedures
are difficult enough when the surveillance involves the use of live and stillborn infants, but
to obtain retrospective data when the event being

examined is an abortion is virtually impossible.
We believe this would be true even if the
occurrence of an abortion was made a reportable
event. Therefore, it is essential that the
information be obtained at the time of the
abortion when important details are fresh in
the minds of the woman and her physician. The
design of the data sheet would be critical;
sufficiently detailed to yield important clues
but compact enough to facilitate rapid collection
of data essential to any monitoring scheme.

 2. Processing of specimens. Deciding on the
nature of the examination of these specimens
might be a difficult matter. However, this particular problem is not peculiar to studies of
embryos and fetuses because in surveillance programmes designed to use live and stillborn data
we know that, as in all studies of large populations, there will be a tremendous variation in
the nature and extent of the examination and
hence in the frequency of detection of defects.
One factor of key importance in any surveillance
scheme is the promptness of reporting, and this
precludes the use of autopsy data in most
instances. Examination of embryos and fetuses
could involve expenditure of considerable time,
but the use of extensive special studies is pro-
hibited if rapid reporting is desirable. Therefore, we believe that the examinations should
involve a survey for external defects, followed
by a simple dissection designed to detect gross
internal malformations. A suggested protocol
is presented in Appendix 1.

 3. Collection of data on anomalous events.
All information on malformations observed in
these abortuses should be forwarded to a
data center where all surveillance information
for a particular region is being examined.

Aside, therefore, from the clerical staff necessary for recording and forwarding data to the central collection office there are two key personnel needed - a person trained in patient interviewing or extraction of relevant data from medical charts (probably a public health nurse) and a pathologist with some training in embryology.

In our opinion the only way of really assessing the costs and the contribution of abortuses to a monitoring system is to establish such a project for a two to three year period, either as a separate programme or preferably as part of an already existing surveillance scheme.

Summary

While it seems reasonable and logical to use embryos and fetuses in any over-all surveillance programme designed to detect new mutagenic and teratogenic agents, there are considerable problems that must be recognized. There are no legal obligations associated with reporting of embryonic and fetal events as there are with live and stillbirths. Although it might be desirable to have abortions as reportable events this is not likely to happen in the very near future. It is obvious, therefore, that only a small percentage of abortuses can be detected and used for study, and there will be a bias in any sample which is used. After considering these biases we believe that spontaneous abortuses are the most useful for purposes of surveillance. Theoretically such abortuses could be included in a monitoring programme with very little difficulty, and it is recommended that a pilot project be established for a two to three year period to evaluate this.

Table 1

Frequency of anomalous abortuses obtained from various sources

SOURCE

	Spontaneous	Ectopic	Induced*	Possibly Induced	Therapeutic
Total	457	21	62	48	94
Abnormal	207	6	9	8	7
% Abnormal	45	35	14	17	7

*Self-induced in most instances but sometimes with non-medical assistance.

APPENDIX

Guide to Post-Mortem Examination
of Embryos and Fetuses

Procedure
   This is based on the method of autopsy performed
on newborns in the Vancouver General Hospital.
Autopsies performed on embryos and fetuses differ,
however, from those performed on newborn infants
chiefly because the embryos are so small that
they do not lend themselves well to gross dissection, and maceration and distortion are much
more common and the latter must be differentiated
from developmental anomaly.

Initial Inspection
   Examination of very small specimens must always
be carried out with the help of a dissecting
microscope. It should also be carried out with
either a picture of a normal or an actual speci-
men present for comparison.
   Inspection - all specimens
Specimen on its back:
   Eyes - eyelids - present - fused.
   Nose - nares - present - patent.
   Lips - complete or cleft.
   Palate - fused or unfused.
   Tongue - size - tip free.
   Neck - evidence of lack of closure or arches.
   Chest
   Cord or body stalk - normal insertion - number
     of vessels.
   Genitalia - genital tubercle, presence of
     vaginal opening.
   Anus - patent or not.
Upper limbs)
) number of rays or digits. Position
Lower limbs)   of hands and feet.

77

Specimen on side:
  position of cleft or ear or pinna with relation
  to angle of jaw.
Specimen on face:
  evidence of non-closure of spinal canal;
  any evidence of swelling or edema in neck;
  any blisters in midline over vertebral column.
All obvious developmental abnormalities should be
either photographed or a drawing should be made
so that a permanent record is made of the anomaly
in that specimen.

Measurements

Crown rump measurements are used in determining
the developmental age of the specimen. This is
correlated with other developmental horizons such
as the development of the eyelids, fusion of
palate, development of digits and presence of
digits and presence of umbilical hernia. The
circumference of the head at the orbital ridges,
circumference of the chest, and circumference of
the neck are taken if the specimen is fresh. The
exact lengths of arm, forearm, head and thigh,
leg and outer border of foot are also taken under
similar circumstances.

Fresh specimens are weighed.

Specimens of 25 mms. or less should then be
placed in 10% formalin in a labelled bottle to
await serial section.

Specimens over 25 mms. should be dissected with
the help of a dissecting microscope when necessary.

The incision should be made slightly to the
left of the cord insertion and continued straight
up towards the chest. The umbilical vein should
be identified and incised where it enters the
liver. The incision is carried around parallel
to the thoracic cage into both loins. Two flaps
can then be pinned back and the contents of the

abdomen exposed.

Identify - check for normality
1. Two umbilical arteries with bladder between them.
2. Appearance of gut.
3. Size of liver.
Raise gut gently and identify gonads, internal genitalia, pancreas. Remove gut by cutting through rectum and gastroduodenal junction, and root of mesentery.
Push down liver and inspect diaphragm.
Dissect out liver.
Identify ureters, kidney and adrenals, spleen, descending aorta and inferior vena cava.

Open the thorax
Make an incision in the midline up as high into the neck as possible and then cut through trachea (above thyroid) and esophagus to vertebral column.
Make an incision around the diaphragm at its insertion into the rib cage. It should now be possible to lift out the thoracic contents, diaphragm and stomach. Incise the abdominal vessels and posterior attachment of the diaphragm and the viscera can then be lifted out of the specimen.
Take a section of trachea which includes thyroid. Lay viscera on dissection board so that esophagus is superior and the upper end towards dissector. Inspect posterior aspect of lungs.
Open esophagus and inspect for possible fistula.
Remove esophagus.
Trachea is now uppermost.
Open trachea to bifuracation.
Turn specimen over.
Identify thymus and remove.
Inspect anterior and lateral aspects of both

lungs.   Remove at roots.
Open pericardium and inspect heart.
Identify pulmonary and aortic trunks, auricles
and ventricles and main veins.

If the heart appears abnormal on inspection do not
dissect.
Open the heart by an incision through the right
auricle parallel to the atrio-ventricular
junction.   Identify foramen ovale.   Incise lateral wall of right ventricle.
Inspect the right ventricle and septum.   Continue incision upwards into pulmonary trunk, to
its termination at the right and left pulmonary
arteries and ductus arteriosis.
On posterior aspect of heart open the left
auricle and identify the atrio-ventricular open-
ing.   Incise left ventricle along its lateral wall
and then up into aorta which may have to be freed
by blunt dissection from pulmonary trunk.
Open aorta over arch and identify branches.
Finally remove one kidney, one adrenal and
spleen from specimen for section.

Thymus
Thyroid
Lung   Are microscopically
Kidney   sectioned where
Adrenal   tissue permits.
Gonad
Spleen
Pancreas

Inspect placenta if present and remove a piece
of amnion which has been fixed in formalin.
Smooth the amnion on a slide and stain for 1 - 2
minutes with buffered Toluidine blue, then cover
with cover slip and squash to flatten as much as
possible.

Examine cells for presence of sex chromatin, and if present do a count of 50 cells. If sex chromatin and phenotypic sex are not compatible, then draw immediate attention to this.
Replace specimen in container.

REFERENCES

1. Newcombe, H.B. Value of Canadian hospital insurance records in detecting increases in congenital anomalies. Canad. Med. Ass. J. 101: 121-128, 1969.
2. Miller, J.R. and Poland, B.J. The value of human abortuses in the surveillance of developmental anomalies. I. General overview. Canad. Med. Ass. J. 103: 501-502, 1970
3. Miller, J.R. and Poland, B.J. The value of human abortuses in the surveillance of developmental anomalies. II. Reduction deformities of the limbs. Canad. Med. Ass. J. 103: 503-505, 1970.
4. Nishimura, H. Fate of human fertilized eggs during prenatal life: present state of knowledge. Okajimas Fol. anal. Jap. 46: 297-305, 1970.
5. Carr, D.H. Chromosome studies in selected spontaneous abortions. I. Conception after oral contraceptives. Canad. Med. Ass. J. 103: 343-348, 1970.
6. Nishimura, H., Takano, K., Tanimura, T. et al. Normal and abnormal development of human embryos. First report of the analysis of 1,213 intact embryos. Teratology 1: 281-290, 1968.

III. MONITORING MAJOR MALFORMATIONS

THE EPIDEMIOLOGY OF THE COMMON MAJOR
MALFORMATIONS AS RELATED TO
ENVIRONMENTAL MONITORING

F. C. Fraser

For the purposes of this paper the "common malformations" will be mostly those in the range of
1/5000 to 1/1000 or so, and will include
anencephaly, spina bifida aperta, club foot,
cleft lip, cleft palate, congenital dislocation
of the hip and pyloric stenosis. They are all
familial, and there is evidence from twins for
most of them that the basis for the familial
distribution is in part genetic. The currently
popular concept of their etiology is that they
result from a developmental process that fails to
reach some sort of threshold. The process if
regulated by a multifactorial system involving
both genes and environmental factors, each with
a relatively small effect. The threshold may be,
for instance, a limiting degree of developmental
unpunctuality, such as failure of the palatal
shelves to reach a horizontal position above the
tongue until it is too late for them to meet and
fuse (Fraser, Walker and Trasler, 1957). The
evidence supporting this concept has been reviewed in a recent WHO report (1970).

In the probably over-simple model proposed by
Falconer (1965), the distribution represents

"liability" to develop the condition in question, and is determined by both genetic and environmental factors; all individuals beyond the threshold are affected. This allows one to estimate heritability from the proportion of affected first degree relatives of probands. More recently, Edwards (1967, 1969) has proposed a model in which the X axis represents the genetic component of liability and the risk of being affected increases exponentially with increasing genetic susceptibility. The latter may be more consistent with reality but the former is easier for the non-mathematically-minded to visualize. Both models lead to fairly high estimates of heritability for the major malformations, but still leave lots of room for environmental variation.

On either model an increase in frequency of the condition would represent either

(1) a shift of the mean towards the threshold, as in the case of first degree relatives of probands, or

(2) an increase in variance, as in the case of parental consanguinity (Newcombe, 1963), or

(3) a shift in the threshold, as in the case of cleft palate; a wide head might require the shelves to become horizontal sooner in order to meet.

Addition of an environmental teratogen, not ubiquitous, to the system would be expected to shift the mean of the distribution in the direction of the threshold, and probably skew the distribution and increase the variance.

We may then ask the question -- "How sensitive an indicator of environmental teratogens are the common malformations likely to be?" And this raises the further questions -- "How good are we at detecting changes in frequency of the common malformations, and what evidence is there that environmental factors do change the frequency?".

I will not consider here the complex problem of getting accurate counts of frequencies except to say that good ascertainment is a prerequisite that is difficult to achieve for many of the major malformations. Frequencies of spontaneous abortion are notoriously difficult to measure. Diagnosis in the neonatal period is unreliable for congenital heart disease, and for dislocation of the hip unless there is careful screening. Pyloric stenosis is not congenital, at least clinically speaking. Club foot shades too gradually into normality. Even cleft palate seems occasionally to get missed, or at least not recorded, in routine reporting systems (Meskin, 1967). We are left, then with three externally obvious and fairly sharply defined conditions: cleft lip, anencephaly and spina bifida aperta, the latter two being etiologically related.

Of these, anencephaly has the poorest evidence for a genetic basis, and the best evidence of sensitivity to environmental factors. It is clearly familial, but there are remarkably few instances of concordant twins except in the series of Gittelsohn and Milham (1965). However, the Falconer model predicts suitably low concordances in MZ twins with heritabilities of 60% or less (Smith, 1970). There is some evidence that the familial tendency is chiefly, if not entirely, maternal (Nance, 1970), though it is still not clear whether this may be accounted for by reporting bias (Carter, 1970). The claim that the frequency is as high in probands' maternal half sibs as it is in their sibs (Yen and Mac-Mahon, 1968) seem to result from an ascertainment bias. Even if anencephaly is caused by cyto-plasmically transmitted agents (Nance, 1970) environmental factors are still important.

There is as much as three-fold variation with socio-economic class in frequency of anenceph-

alics (eight-fole in stillborns) demonstrated in
several populations (Edwards, 1958; Williamson,
1965; Naggan and MacMahon, 1967; Horowitz and
McDonald, 1969). This does not correlate with
illegitimacy (Edwards, 1958) and seems unlikely
to be due to genetic differences in socio-economic status.

A seasonal fluctuation of up to three-fold,
with an excess in the winter months, has been
reported for Scotland in 1939-1955 (reviewed by
Edwards, 1958), the United Kingdon in 1954-1960
(Slater et al., 1964), Birmingham from 1945 to
1956 (Edwards, 1961), and Germany in 1950-1961
(Tünte, 1968), but not in Rhode Island in 1936-
1952 (MacMahon et al., 1953), in France in 1945-
1955 (Frézal et al., 1954), in Liverpool in
1960-1962 (Smithells, 1964) or in Quebec in 1956-
1965 (Horowitz and McDonald, 1969). This geographic variation in seasonal variation led
Edwards (1964) to propose the "deep-freeze
hypothesis" -- namely that modern methods of
storing foods are removing seasonal fluctuation
in some dietary factor. Other hypotheses can be
imagined but, whatever the relevant factor is,
we may never find it, as it seems to be dis-
appearing.

There are also secular trends. The frequency
of anencephaly fell in New York State from 1945-
1959 (Gittelsohn and Milham, 1962) and in New
England from 1946 to 1965 (Naggan and MacMahon,
1967), but not in South Wales from 1956-1965
(Lawrence et al., 1968). In Birmingham it fell
from 1940 to 1949, rose until 1956 and then fell
again (Leck, 1966). Why?

Marked regional variations occur (Lilienfeld,
1970). Lowest frequencies are reported from
Israel (0.6 per 1000 births) and highest from
Ireland (4.6/1000). There are curious gradients
in frequency, decreasing from West to East

in Europe (Penrose, 1957) but from East to West
in South Wales (Lawrence et al., 1968) and
probably Canada (Horowitz and McDonald, 1969).
Urban rates seem to be higher than rural rates in
Northamptonshire (Pleydell, 1960), in Quebec
(Horowitz and McDonald, 1969) and probably South
Wales (Lawrence et al., 1968). These may reflect
genetic and socio-economic differences, variations in maternal age and parity (Record, 1961),
or variations in reporting practice, etc., but
they may also represent relevant environmental
variables. Correlations have been reported, for
instance, with rainfall in Holland (Rootselaar,
1967) but not South Wales (Lawrence et al.,1963),
with Asian influenza (Coffey and Jessop, 1957;
Pleydell, 1960), with decrease in height of
mother (Anderson et al., 1958) and with background radiation (Gentry, 1959), and cosmic
radiation (Wesley, 1960), though the latter
claims have been discredited (Grahn and Kratchman, 1963; Spiers et al., 1960; Hewitt, 1963).

One is repeatedly tantalized by reports of
clustering of anencephaly and other malformations
(Pleydell, 1960; Lucy, 1964; Flynt, 1970); that
is, short term variations in incidence in specific regions. Attempts to identify relevant factor
factors have so far been highly unsuccessful. We
need better reporting systems to identify such
clusters quickly, and some sort of protocol for
investigating them, with perhaps a center that
could coordinate such studies, do the appropriate
tests and even send a team to the "epidemic"
area (Miller, 1970).

It should be emphasized that most, if not all
of the variables discussed so far may well represent "normal" variations in our environment
rather than the presence of specific teratogens.
This does not detract from the importance of
counting them, but emphasizes that the main

reason for their surveillance is to identify the relevant variables, with a view to reducing the frequency of these major sources of ill-health, rather than to monitor the environment for new teratogens.

Racial variations may represent another approach to the detection of environmental variations (Carter, 1970). Anencephaly is infrequent in oriental races (Stevenson et al.,1966) and Jews, both in Israel (Halevi, 1967), the eastern United States (Haggan and MacMahon, 1967) and Quebec (Horowitz and McDonald, 1969). The low frequency in Jews may account for some of the previously mentioned regional (e.g. urban-rural) and social class differences. Anencephaly is strikingly high in Sikhs, both in the Punjab (Carter, 1970) and in Bombay (Searle, 1959). In Boston the frequency in the Irish decreased with the number of generations since emigration (Naggan and MacMahon, 1967). In Quebec the "French-Canadian" rate was higher than that in France but lower than that in Britain. These changes seem more likely to represent changing environments than miscegenation, but what are the relevant variables?

It follows from the multifactorial-threshold model that in conditions appearing more often in one sex than the other, the sex ratio should change as the population frequency changes. Anencephaly occurs much more often in females than in males, and one should expect an increase in sex ratio in populations with a high frequency of anencephaly. Just how much of an increase depends on which model one chooses, and what assumptions are made about the relative effects of environmental factors in the two sexes. It would be interesting to see what the sex ratio is in the sibs of probands, a population with a high incidence. From the small amount of data available, the sex ratio does not appear to increase (Williamson, 1965; Carter et al., 1968).

Possible changes in sex ratio of appropriate malformations might be a more sensitive indicator of changing frequency than direct counts, and at least they might serve to indicate whether reported changes in frequency are real or simply represent reporting bias. Unfortunately, in the case of anencephaly, the situation is complicated by the fact that the sex ratio increases with length of gestation, suggesting that female anencephalics have a higher prenatal mortality, and making comparisons between series tenuous. The sex ratio is low for whites in New York State but high for negroes, which supports the hypothesis, (since negroes have the lower frequency) on the basis of the Falconer model. It might be worth while looking into this for other malformations with aberrant sex ratios.

Other common malformations also show the kind of variations described above (Lilienfeld, 1970; Carter, 1970). None has shown as many environmental associations as anencephaly, but this may be due in part to a less intensive search. My comments are relevant to them also.

Another common "malformation" that might be worth considering is heterochromia iridis, though this would probably need to be done some months after birth. In children exposed to intrauterine X-radiation in the first five months of gestation, 8/567 or 1.4% had a sector of the iris different in color from the rest, as compared to 3 of 3972 or 0.07% in the controls (Lejeune et al., 1961).

These might result from somatic mutations or non-genetic developmental damage. In either case, an increase would be disquieting.

Finally, from what is known of teratogens in experimental animals and from the few recognized in man, one might expect that a new environmental teratogen would cause an increase in multiple malformations. It would therefore be useful to count the proportion of anencephalics that have other major malformations, and similarly for cleft lip, cleft palate and so on. This would also be subject to the usual reporting biases, but probably not so much as the malformations counted singly. Furthermore, since multiple malformations are a fairly small portion of the total, an increase in these would be a fairly small increase in frequency of each malformation counted singly but would be a proportionately bigger increase in the multiple group -- that is, the effect would be magnified by considering the multiple malformations separately.

In conclusion, monitoring major malformations is desirable in order to identify relevant environmental factors, with the hope of prevention. This will require improvements in our methods of counting, and some mechanism for initiating ad hoc studies when and where indicated. Changes in sex ratio deserve further attention in conditions with aberrant sex ratios. As an indicator of new environmental teratogens, surveillance for an increase in multiple malformations would probably be more sensitive than counting individual malformations.

REFERENCES

Banister, P. Congenital malformations: preliminary report of an investigation of reduction deformities of the limbs, triggered by a surveillance system. Can. Med. Assoc. J. 103: 466-472, 1970.

Carter, C.O., David, P.A. and Laurence, K.M. A family study of major central nervous system malformations in South Wales. J. Med. Gen. 5 (2): 81-106, 1968.

Carter, C.O. Multifactorial inheritance revisited. In "Congenital Malformations". F.C. Fraser and V. McKusick, Eds., Excerpta Medica, New York, 1970, pp. 227-232.

Edwards, J.H. Congenital malformations of the central nervous system in Scotland. Brit. J. Prev. Soc. Med. 12(3): 115-130, 1958.

Edwards, J.H. Seasonal incidence of congenital disease in Birmingham. Ann. Hum. Gen. 25: 89-93, 1961.

Edwards, J.H. The epidemiology of congenital malformations. Proc. 2nd Intern. Conf. on Cong. Malf. pp. 297-305, 1963.

Edwards, J.H. Linkage studies of whole populations. Proc. 3rd Intern. Cong. of Human Genetics. Plenary Sessions and Symposia. The Johns Hopkins Press, Baltimore, 1967, pp. 479-482.

Edwards, J.H. Familial predisposition in man. Brit. Med. Bull. 25(1): 58-64, 1969.

Falconer, D.S. The inheritance of liability to certain diseases, estimated from the incidence among relatives. Ann. Hum. Gen. 29(1): 51-71, 1965.

Flynt, J.W. An unusual incidence of central nervous system defects in a military population (Abst.). Teratology 3(2): 199-200, 1970.

Fraser, F.C., Walker, B.E. and Trasler, D.G. Experimental production of congenital cleft palate: genetic and environmental factors. Pediatrics 19(No. 4, part II): 782-787, 1957.

Frezal, J., Kelly, J., Guillemot, M.L. and Lamy, M. Anencephaly in France. Amer. J. Hum. Gen. 16(3): 336-350, 1964.

Gittelsohn, A. M., and Milham, S. Declining incidence of central nervous system anomalies in New York State. Brit. J. Prev. Soc. Med. 16: 153, 1962.

Gittelsohn, A.M., and Milham, S. Vital record

incidence of congenital malformations in New York State in "Genetics and the epidemiology of chronic diseases." Neel, J.V., Shaw, M.W. and Schull, W.J. Eds. United States Department of Health Education and Welfare, Public Health Science Publication 1163 1965, 305.

Grahn, D. and Kratchman, J. Variation if neonatal death rate and birth weight in the U United States and possible relations to environmental radiation, geology and altitude. Amer. J. Hum. Gen. 15(4): 329-352, 1963.

Halevi, H.S. Congenital malformations in Israel. Brit. J. Prev. Soc. Med. 21: 66-67, 1967.

Hewitt, D. Geographical variations in the mortality attributed to spina bifida and other congenital malformations. Brit. J. Prev. Soc. Med. 17(1): 13-22, 1963.

Horowitz, I. and McDonald, A.D. Anencephaly and spina bifida in the Province of Quebec. Can. Med. Assoc. J. 100: 748-755, 1969.

Laurence, K.M., Carter, C.O. and David, P.A. Major central nervous system malformations in South Wales. Brit. J. Prev. Soc. Med. 22(3): 146-160, 1968.

Leck, I. Changes in the incidence of neural tube defects. Lancet II: 791-793, 1966.

Lejeune, J., Turpin, R. and Rethore, M.O. Les effets somatiques de l'irradiation du goetus in utero. Therapie 16: 521-529, 1961.

Lilienfeld, A.M. Population differences in frequency of malformations at birth. In "Congenital Malformations". F.C. Fraser and V. McKusick, Eds., Excerpta Medica, New York, 1970, pp. 251-263.

Lucy, J.F., Mann, R.W., Simmons, G.M., and Friedman, E. An increased incidence of spina bifida in Vermont in 1962. Pediatrics 33 (6): 981-984, 1964.

MacMahon, B., Pugh. T.F. and Ingalls, T.H. Anencephalus, spina bifida, and hydrocephalus incidence related to sex, race, and season of birth, and incidence in siblings. Brit. J. Prev. Soc. Med. 7(4): 211-219, 1953.

Meskin, L.H. and Pruzansky, S. Validity of the birth certificate in the epidemiologic assessment of facial clefts. J. Dent. Res. 46(6) Pt. 2: 1456-1459, 1967.

Miller, R.W. Teratology in 1970: The National Scene. President's Report to the Teratology Society. Teratology 3(3): 223-227, 1970.

Naggan, L. and MacMahon, B. Ethnic differences in the prevalence of anencephaly and spina bifida in Boston, Massachusetts. New England J. Med. 277: 1119-1123, 1967.

Nance, W.E. Anencephaly and spina bifida: a possible example of cytoplasmic inheritance in man. Nature 224: 373-375, 1969.

Newcombe, H.B. The phenodeviant theory. In "Congenital Malformations" M. Fishbein, Ed., International Medical Congress Limited, New York, 1963, pp. 345-349.

Penrose, L.S. Genetics of anencephaly. J. Ment. Def. Res. 1(1): 4-15, 1957.

Pleydell, M.J. Anencephaly and other congenital abnormalities. An epidemiological study in Northamptonshire. Brit. Med. J. 1: 309-314, 1960.

Record, R.G. Anencephalus in Scotland. Brit. Med. J. Prev. Soc. Med. 15 93-105, 1961.

Rootselaar, F.J. van, and Beks, J.W.F. Spina bifida and anencephaly in Holland 1950-1963. An epidemiological model. Develop. Med. Child Neurol. (Cited by Laurence et al., 1968).

Searle, A.G. The incidence of anencephaly in a polytypic population. Ann Eugen. 23 (3): 279-288, 1959.

Slater, B.C.S., Watson, G. I., and McDonald, J.C. Seasonal variation in congenital abnormal-

J.C. Seasonal variation in congenital abnormalities: preliminary report of a survey conducted by the Research Committee of the Council of the College of General Practitioners. Brit. J. Prev. Soc. Med. 18 (1): 1-7, 1964.

Smith, C. Heritability of liability and concordance in monozygous twins. Ann. Hum. Gen. 34: 85-91, 1970.

Smithells, R.W., Chinn, E.R. and Franklin, D. Anencephaly in Liverpool. Dev. Med. and Child Neurol. 6(3): 231-240, 1964.

Spiers, F.W., Burch, P.R.J. and Reed, G.W. Background radiation as the cause of fatal congenital malformation. Int. J. Rad. Biol. 2: 235-236, 1960.

Tunte, W. Zur Haufigkeit angeborener Missbildungen des Zentralnervensystems und des Verdauungstraktes in der Jahren 1950-1961. Humangenetik 6: 29-33, 1968.

Wesley, J.P. Background radiation as the cause of fatal congenital malformation. Intern. J. Rad. Biol. 2(1): 97-118, 1960.

Williamson, E.M. Incidence and family aggregation of major congenital malformations of central nervous system. J. Med. Gen. 2(3): 161-172, 1965.

World Health Organization. Genetic factors in congenital malformations. WHO Technical Report Series No. 438, 1970.

STUDIES IN CHILDHOOD CANCER AS A GUIDE FOR MONITORING CONGENITAL MALFORMATIONS

Robert W. Miller

Cancer

It is easier at present to monitor for cancer than for congenital malformations. One might expect the reverse to be true because there are about 120,000 new cases of major congenital malformations each year in the United States as compared with about 5,000 new cancer cases under 15 years of age. The much greater lethality of cancer, however, simplifies the ascertainment of cases. In consequence, death certificates are an effective data resource for research into cancer. Astonishing differences between comparison groups may be revealed by such study. Only recently, for example, was the rarity of Ewing's tumor in the Negro discovered by review of U.S. national mortality from bone cancer among children (1-3). This is the kind of finding that is unlikely to be made by physicians on the basis of their clinical experience, or from a review of hospital charts. Also unrecognizable except at the national level is the two-fold greater mortality from retinoblastoma among Negroes as compared with Whites

Congenital Malformations

Because congenital malformations are often not lethal, death certificates can be used only to a small extent as a monitoring device. A serious

handicap in the use of routinely coded death-
certificate diagnosis is insufficient detail in
the coding system used (International Classification of Disease and Causes of Death[5]).
Diagnoses are often grouped in a fashion that is
unsatisfactory for research purposes. We have
gotten around this problem in cancer studies by
securing copies of death certificates for all
children who died of cancer in the United States,
beginning in 1960 and continuing thus far through
1967. Each diagnosis has been re-coded as to
cell type through use of the systematized Nomenclature of Pathology[6]. The amount of new
information available from this resource has been
immense. To give but one example: by coding the
mother's maiden name, which is supposed to be
entered on all death certificates and actually is
recorded on a high proportion, we have been able
to identify twins and other sibs who have died of
cancer during the interval under study. (Through
the use of alphabetized lists, sibs were identified primarily by matching surnames and mothers'
maiden names.) In consequence, it was possible
to improve the estimate of the concordance rate
for leukemia in presumably identical twins, and
to demonstrate that the concordance fades with
age and has virtually disappeared by 6 years.
The death certificates have also established that
sibs of children with fatal brain cancer have 9
times the usual risk of dying from this neoplasm,
and, a totally unexpected finding, they also have
9 times the usual risk of dying from cancer of
the bone or muscle.[7,8]

The same sort of death-certificate registry
could be established for congenital malformations. For some anomalies difficulties in interpreting the results may be expected, because
mortality is, of course, influenced by therapy
and by fluctuations in the frequency of superim-

posed lethal infections. The accuracy in recording diagnoses of congenital malformations on death certificates may vary considerably with the type of malformation and from one locale to another. Tabulations of the frequencies of fatal malformations will lag several years behind the dates of death. Nevertheless, it would be useful to make a national study of data not routinely coded from death certificates concerning malformations that were lethal within the first 28 days of life, and perhaps throughout infancy.

Fetal Death

Post-natal observations are, of course, not the only measures of teratogenesis. In those areas where fetal death certificates are of better than average quality the frequency and causes of such mortality can be evaluated. One could look within states for sharp increases in the numbers of such occurrences over time. Again, a substantial lag would occur before unusual fluctuations in frequencies from these routinely processed vital certificates could be determined. Yet, if the results proved of interest, ways to shorten and otherwise improve the procedure might be devised.

BIRTH CERTIFICATES

In a large number of states the birth certificate contains an item under which congenital malformations may be recorded. The extent to which an entry is made here varies with the detectability of malformations at birth and the conscientiousness of the physician who signs the birth certificate. Even if the anomaly is unmistakable and is properly recorded, the effort is to no avail in most states; the item is not coded. In consequence, there is no rapid way in which affected children may be identified. A select committee convened by the National Center for Health Statistics has recommended[9] that efforts be made to improve and use data concerning congenital malformations recorded on birth certificates, but no attempt has been made to implement this recommendation.

HOSPITAL RECORDS

Cancer

Individual clinical observations and hospital records have been a valuable source of information concerning characteristics of children with cancer. Physicians at the bedside or in the clinic may gain important new understanding of etiology from the history or physical findings of a single case or a small series of cases. It was in this way that the increased occurrence of leukemia in Down's syndrome was first suspected.[10] Recognition of an epidemic of respiratory cancer among Japanese mustard-gas workers began with an intern asking a 30-year-old man why he had lung cancer at such an early age.[11]

Congenital Malformations

The chances for recognizing new teratogenic agents would be enhanced if physicians were to ask about and record the mother's occupation and unusual environmental exposures just before or during the relevant pregnancy. Teratologic research would also be aided if anomalies incidentally found during the medical examination were not buried in scribbled entries under the organ system involved, but were also listed under the diagnoses made at the end of the admission record, on the face-sheet of the chart, and, when death occurs, on the death certificate in the space provided for other significant diseases.

REGISTRIES AND SCREENING STUDIES

Cancer

Cancer registries have been established in various areas of the world, including a substantial number of developing countries.[12] Registry data have been used for occasional studies of morbidity, clustering and the outcome of therapy. Far more use of data can be made.

Congenital malformations

Registries for congenital malformations are uncommon. It is difficult to establish an effective system on reports submitted by physicians and hospitals throughout an area. The effort involved is huge and often focuses more on collecting data than analyzing it. One system, more successful than most, is the Registry for Handicapped Children and Adults in British Columbia, Canada. From his experience with this registry, Dr. James R. Miller [13] has advised that "routine documentation (of congenital malformations) . . . to be used effectively. . . must be linked with routine vital and health statistics."

In the United States, the Metropolitan Atlanta Congenital Defects Program has collected data on major malformations observed at birth in the hospitals of the 5-county area under study. The sponsors of the Program issue tabulations monthly.[14] Since October 1967 when the surveillance began, there has been no cluster of specific anomalies to suggest the influence of an environmental agent.

Screening programs are far more common than registries for congenital malformations. These programs involve standard examination of infants or young children in a single hospital (e.g. Columbia University Fetal Life Study[15]) in prepaid hospital systems (e.g. Kaiser-Permanente[16] and the Health Insurance Plan of Greater New York[17]), in geographically scattered collaborating hospitals (Collaborative Perinatal Research Program of the National Institute of Neurological Diseases and Stroke, NIH[18]), in a multihospital audit system that covers millions of people (Commission on Professional Hospital Activities, Ann Arbor, Michigan), and all the hospitals in a metropolitan area (Birmingham, England[19]). All lagged far behind in looking for time trends. Furthermore, no new environmental agent has been found by any of these studies to be teratogenic. In fact, the NINDS Collaborative Study could not detect by clinical examination alone the epidemic of rubella embryopathy that occurred in the United States in 1964.[20] The greatest asset of this Program was the blood samples drawn from mothers during pregnancy and from cord blood. Virologic study of these samples has produced new understanding of the more subtle effects from teratogenic microbial agents.[21] The relationship between the outcome of pregnancy and specific drug therapy of the mother has been evaluated by the Kaiser-Permanente group[22] and in the Columbia Fetal Life Study[23] but, on the whole, the cost and effort of these large-scale endeavors has not been commensurate with the new information developed.

Surveillance of congenital malformations at birth has also been made on an international scale. Under the sponsorship of the World Health Organization, Stevenson, et al[24,25] collected data on malformations at 24 centers in 16 countries. Some of the results were strange. For example, among about 66,000 Indian births, none were reported to have Down's Syndrome. Among the 24 centers the rates for 1,000 total births ranged from 0.00 to 3.89 (standardized for maternal age). Recently, Stevenson[26] has expressed the opinion that the study contributed "relatively little to our understanding of comparative frequencies." He felt that the international study in conjunction with other national studies suggested "the need for more careful ad hoc epidemiological studies of individual malformations . . . (and) that much good use can be made of . . . pre-recorded data."

Ponderous epidemiologic methods are valid, but no major human teratogen has been recognized in this way. Malformations induced by X-ray, German measles, thalidomide and organic mercury (congenital Minamata disease) were each recognized by an alert practitioner who observed a cluster of cases and then traced the disease to its source. Such episodes in the future will probably be recognized as they were in the past -- by medical specialists to whom children with specific defects are referred for therapy. The specialist represents a point of concentration for such patients.

To enhance recognition of sudden changes in malformation rates, a systematic collection of data from concentration points should be established. Specifically, a surveillance should be made, if possible, of claims submitted to private, state, or local agencies for the medical care of children with birth defects. Feasibility studies in several states as well as in certain Canadian provinces may lead to larger scale coverage. Such a system, though less complete than cancer registries, may be easier to establish over a large area, and may be of greater value in etiologic research.

INTERNATIONAL ORGANIZATIONS

The best evidence for a virus in childhood

oncogenesis comes from an international comparison that revealed a very high frequency of Burkitt's lyphoma in Central Africa. With a grant of only $400 for an ancient station wagon, Dr. Burkitt determined the geographic boundaries beyond which the neoplasm did not occur. Since then tremendous resources have been poured into the study of the tumor. By contrast, virtually no interest was shown in congenital Minamata disease until pollution of water with organic mercury was recently found to be a potential problem in the United States.

Oncology is much more international than teratology is. There are two very active international organizations entirely devoted to cancer research. The International Union Against Cancer has standing committees to promote interest and an exchange of ideas among nations. The other organization, the International Agency for Research on Cancer, conducts epidemiologic research. There are no counterparts in teratology. A first step would be the establishment of a committee by the Internal Congress on Congenital Malformations to encourage the fullest possible study of accidental or industrial exposures to substantial doses of potential teratogens (e.g. pesticides or defoliants) during pregnancy. The Committee might stand ready to assist in the evaluation of exceptional exposures wherever in the world they occurred.

OCCUPATIONAL STUDIES

Occupational studies have yielded a large array of exposures that cause cancer in man.[27] For teratologic research, there is a need to explore the availability of data in various countries concerning industrial exposures during pregnancy that may have an adverse effect on the embryo.

TIME-SPACE CLUSTERS

With excitement over the possibility that human cancer may be induced by viruses, there has been great interest in the occurrence of individual clusters of specific forms of cancer within certain communitites. In none of the studies has an agent been identified or even brought under suspicion. Chance may still explain all of the occurrences reported to date. The question really is not do clusters occur, but do they occur excessively? To this end, several statisticians have invented techniques to determine if rare events, such as specific categories of cancer, cluster excessively in time and space.[28] These techniques involve the dispassionate evaluation of the distribution of cases with respect to sub-units of the geographic area and the time-interval under study. The procedure is applicable not only to cancer but to any rare event, such as the births of children with Down's syndrome. (When applied to that particular anomaly in a series of about 2,500 cases, the statistical test revealed no excessive clustering.[29]) The procedure requires, however, unbiased ascertainment of cases, and for this reason its use in studying most forms of congenital malformations is at present very limited.

RECORD-LINKAGE

Cancer

In an evaluation of cancer mortality among steelworkers, more than 30 steps were involved in tracing the subjects from employment to death. To locate people after intervals of years, it is conventional to consult among others, credit

105

agencies, the police, neighbors and relatives. To complete one such study requires one full-time epidemiologist or statistician assisted by a half-dozen clerks over an interval of 3-5 years. Only a few studies of this nature can be undertaken by a scientist in a life-time.

Several countries are well ahead of the United States in establishing record-linkage systems for health studies.[30] Acheson in Great Britain has been at the forefront. The United States has several resources which permit record-linkage for certain sub-groups of the population. One of the most notable involves the Follow-up Agency of the National Academy of Sciences-National Research Council. The Agency has access to the military service and veterans' records of about 30 million men who have served in the Armed Forces since World War I (1917).[31] Military exposures can be related to causes of death of the subject, or causes of death can be related to military exposures. In this instance, use is made of death certificates which are filed with the Veterans Administration by a very high proportion of survivors to support claims for burial benefits. Paternal exposures in relation to the health of offspring can be determined through mail questionaires,[32] but most studies through the use of this resource have concerned the health of the veterans themselves.

Congenital Malformations

Follow-up studies and investigations into health aspects of mother and child, and among sibs or other close relatives are greatly aided by record-linkage. Systems for those purposes are rare in the United States. The Kaiser-Permanente prepaid medical program has the capability, but it has not yet been well developed. In Canada, Newcombe[33] has been active in such

studies. Opportunities for research of this
nature in the United States would be substantially
increased if the child were given a social security number at birth, which along with the mother's
social security number could be routinely recorded on hospital and vital records of the child.
This procedure would make record-linkage possible
through the use of computers, and immensely
reduce the time and personnel that would otherwise be required.

VETERINARY STUDIES

Cancer

Finally, study of cancer in domestic animals
may provide clues to human oncogenesis. The
observation that giant breeds of dogs (such as
St. Bernard and Great Dane) have about 200 times
the relative frequency of bone cancer that small
and medium size dogs have[34] suggests that rate of
bone growth within a species is a determinant of
this form of neoplasia.

Congenital Malformations

In teratogenesis, the value of observations in
domestic and wild animals was exemplified in the
study of Minamata disease. Identification of
mercury-contaminated fish as the source of the
epidemic was aided by noting that cats and birds
that ate the fish developed neurologic disorders.
More recently, a brief report published in the
December 1969 issue of Modern Veterinary Practice
described epidemics of lethal skeletal deformities among pigs on 5 farms in central Kentucky
over a 2-year period. The author called attention
to the fact that during pregnancy the pigs had
access to tobacco stalks that had been sprayed
with chemicals including growth regulants to control suckering, and various insecticides.

whether or not these occurrences, of potentially great clinical importance, have been more fully investigated, I do not know.

CONCLUSION

In perspective, it appears that cancer epidemiology may serve as a guide to a variety of studies that could be made with respect to congenital malformations. What is needed primarily, however, is a scientific group at the national level to make the most of existing resources to this end.

REFERENCES

1. Fraumeni, J.F., Jr. and Glass, A.G.: Rarity of Ewing's sarcoma among U.S. Negro children. Lancet 1: 366-367, 1970.
2. Jensen, R.D. and Drake, R.M.: Rarity of Ewing's tumor in Negroes. Lancet 1: 777, 1970.
3. Linden, G. and Dunn, J.E.: Ewing's sarcoma in Negroes. Lancet 1: 1171, 1970.
4. Jensen, R.D. and Miller, R.W.: To be published.
5. Manual of the International Statistical Classification of Diseases, Injuries, and Causes of Death, ed. 7, Geneva, Switzerland, 1957, World Health Organization.
6. Systematized Nomenclature of Pathology, ed.1, Chicago, 1965, College of American Pathologists.
7. Miller, R.W.: Deaths from childhood cancer in sibs. New Eng. J. Med. 279: 122-126, 1968.
8. Miller, R.W.: Deaths from childhood leukemia and solid tumors among twins and other sibs in the United States, 1960-67. J. Nat. Cancer Inst. In press.
9. Vital and Health Statistics, Documents and Committee Reports: Use of Vital and Health Records in Epidemiologic Research. A report of

the United States National Committee on Vital and Health Statistics. Public Health Service Publication No. 1000, Series 4, No. 7, 1968.

10. Bernard, J., Mathé, G., and Delorme, J-Cl.: Les leucoses des trés jeunes enfants. Arch. Franc. Pediat. 12:470-502, 1954.

11. Miller, R.W.: Environmental agents in cancer. Yale J. Biol. Med. 37: 487-502, 1965.

12. Doll, R., Payne, P., and Waterhouse, J.: Cancer Incidence in Five Continents. A Technical Report. New York, 1966, Springer-Verlag.

13. Miller, J.R.: The use of a registry for the study of congenital defect. In: Nishimura, H. and Miller, J.R. (Eds.): Methods for Teratological Studies in Experimental Animals and Man. Tokyo, Japan, Igaku Shoin Ltd. 1969, pp. 206-214.

14. Metropolitan Atlanta Congenital Defects Program: Monthly reports issued by the National Chronic Disease Center, Atlanta, Georgia.

15. Mellin, G.W.: The fetal life study of the Columbia Presbyterian Medical Center. In Chipman, S.S., Lilienfeld, A.M., Greenberg, B.G., and Donnelly, J.F. (Eds.): Research Methodology and Needs in Perinatal Studies. Springfield, Illinois, 1966, Charles C. Thomas, pp.88-103.

16. Van den Berg, B.J.: Morbidity of low birth weight and/or preterm children compared to that of the "mature". I. Methodological considerations and findings for the first 2 years of life. Pediatrics 42: 590-597, 1968.

17. Shapiro, S.: Methodology in the study of pregnancy outcome and childhood disorders being conducted by the Health Insurance Plan. In Chipman, S.S., Lilienfeld, A.M., Greenberg, B. G., and Donnelly, J.F. (Eds.): Research Methodology and Needs in Perinatal Studies. Springfield, Illinois, 1966, Charles C. Thomas , pp. 39-57.

18. Berendes, H.W.: The structure and scope of the collaborative project on cerebral palsy,

mental retardation, and other neurological and
sensory disorders of infancy and childhood. In
Chipmann, S.S., Lilienfeld, A.M., Greenberg, B.G.
and Donnelly, J.F. (Eds.): Research Methodology
and Needs in Perinatal Studies. Springfield,
Illinois, 1966, Charles C. Thomas, pp.118-138.
19. Leck, I., Record, R.G., McKeown, T. and
Edwards, J.H.: The incidence of malformations in
Birmingham, England, 1950-1959. Teratology 1:
263-280, 1968.
20. Sever, J.L., Nelson, K.B., and Gilkeson,
M.R.: Rubella epidemic, 1964: effect on 6,000
pregnancies. I. Preliminary clinical and laboratory findings through the neonatal period: a
report from the collaborative study on cerebral
palsy. Amer. J. Dis. Child. 110: 395-407, 1965.
21. Sever, J.L.: Perinatal infections affecting
the developing fetus and newborn. In: The
Prevention of Mental Retardation through Control
of Infectious Diseases. U.S. Department of
Health, Education and Welfare, Public Health
Service, Publication No. 1962, Washington, D.C.,
U.S. Government Printing Office, 1968, pp. 37-68.
22. Yerushalmy, J. and Milkovich, L.: Evaluation of the teratogenic effect of meclizine in
man. Amer. J. Obstet. Gynec. 93: 553-562, 1965.
23. Mellin, G.W.: Drugs in the first trimester
of pregnancy and the fetal life of Homo sapiens.
Amer. J. Obstet. Gynec. 90: 1169-1180, 1964.
24. Stevenson, A.C., Johnston, H.A., Stewart,
M.I.P. and Golding, D.R.: Congenital malformations: A report of a study of series of consecutive births in 24 centres. Bull, WHO, Suppl.
Vol. 34, 1966.
25. Stevenson, A.C., Johnston, H.A., Stewart,
M.I.P. and Golding D.R.: Comparative Study of
Congenital Malformations. Basic Tabulations in
Respect of Consecutive Post 28-week Births Recorded in Co-operating Centres. Medical Research

Council, Population Genetics Research Unit, Oxford, 1966.

26. Stevenson, A.C.: Findings and lessons for the future from a comparative study of congenital malformations at 24 centres in 16 countries: In Nishimura, H. and Miller, J.R. (Eds.): Methods for Teratological Studies in Experimental Animals and Man. Tokyo, Japan, Igaku Shoin Ltd. 1969, pp. 195-205.

27. Doll, R.: Prevention of Cancer. Pointers from Epidemiology. London, 1967, The Nuffield Provincial Hospitals Trust.

28. Mantel, N.: The detention of disease clustering and a generalized regression approach. Cancer Res. 27: 209-220, 1967.

29. Stark, C.R. and Mantel, N.: Lack of seasonal or temporal-spatial clustering of Down's Syndrome births in Michigan. Amer. J. Epid. 86: 199-213, 1967.

30. Acheson, E.D.: Record-linkage in Medicine. Proceedings of the International Symposium. Oxford, July 1967. Baltimore, 1968, Williams and Wilkins Company.

31. DeBakey, M.E. and Beebe, G.W.: Medical follow-up studies on veterans. J.A.M.A. 182: 1103-1109, 1962.

32. Miller, R.W. and Jablon, S.: A search for late radiation effects among men who served as X-ray technologists in the U.S. Army during World War II. Radiology 96: 335-359, 1967.

34. Tjalma, R.A.: Canine bone sarcoma: estimation of relative risk as a function of body size. J. Nat. Cancer Inst. 36: 1137-1150, 1966.

DISCUSSION

DR. HOOK: I'd like to ask Dr. Robert Miller to make some comments on monitoring for radiation, in view of the well known susceptibility of irradiated fetuses to develop tumors later in their lifetime. Do you feel that tumors would be useful markers of radiation surveillance and, if not, what other markers -- sex ratio, perinatal mortality, microcephaly, fetal wastage or prematurity -- would be useful in a general scheme specifically devoted to radiation?

DR. R. MILLER: If the dose is high, small head circumference with mental retardation would be the best indicator, as revealed by the studies in Japan. If the woman was early in pregnancy and close enough to the hypocenter, almost all children had these defects. No other malformations have been observed in the group study at Hiroshima. If you're speaking of low-dose exposures, as I think you are, the sex ratio certainly is too insensitive and too difficult to use. Small head circumference and other defects would not be helpful. The occurrence of tumors and leukemia, on theoretical grounds, might be what one would look for the most. However, Alice Stewart and Dr. MacMahon of Boston have both shown that all tumors of children are equally increased in frequency when the mothers receive very small doses of x-ray for diagnostic purposes during pregnancy. The question is whether or not it makes sense that all tumors would be equally induced by such "homeopathic" radiation dosage. The data, and the people who collected it, are excellent. The problem is the explanation. Is it really the radiation or is it something else that explains the increase in tumor occurrence under ten years of age? Dr. Stewart has recently

published an estimate of the number of increased
tumors that would be expected if each of a million children received one rad during intrauterine life -- and she estimated that a million-
person rads received in utero will produce 300 to
800 extra cancer deaths under ten years of age.

DR. SMITH: Dr. Fraser, would you comment on
the sex ratio in anencephaly in abortuses as compared to more full term anencephaly. Is there
good data on that?

DR. FRASER: Not to my knowledge. I checked
the literature and couldn't find anything on sex-
ratio in anencephalies aborted early in pregnancy.

DR. HOOK: Dr. Fraser, how less useful would it
be to pool the three main CNS malformations
(spina bifida, hydrocephaly and anencephaly) together in a monitoring scheme searching for
environmental effects, at least in the first
analysis?
   Secondly, in view of the well known open type
request for congenital malformations on birth
certificates, the recording is markedly variable.
In view of that, however, and in view of the fact
that cleft lip and some of the CNS defects are
the best markers, would it not be valuable to
urge a change in certificates, asking a specific
question on the certificate about these two types
of defects?

DR. FRASER: As far as the first question goes,
I think there has been a great deal of confusion
caused by pooling hydrocephalus, anencephalus and
spina bifida, because much of the hydrocephalus
is related anatomically to the spina bifida and
yet there are many cases of hydrocephalus that
have nothing to do with spina bifida. The early

literature at least, does lump many of these and one gets misleading results thereby, so I would urge <u>not</u> pooling from that point of view. Furthermore, I think one might learn a good deal about the genetics and embryology of the anencephaly and sex ratios independently. In other words, it would be useful to have anencephaly <u>without</u> spina bifida, anencephaly <u>with</u> spina bifida and spina bifida <u>without</u> anencephaly recorded separately. Then we might start to make some sense of the multifactorial model. Without such data it is very difficult.

DR. R. MILLER: With regard to the question of whether or not specific malformations should have a check list on the birth certificate, that recommendation was made by the same expert committee whose pamphlet I mentioned.

DR. FRASER: Would you recommend substituting these two malformations?

DR. R. MILLER: No. I think there should be selected questions, not necessarily just two but whatever number was thought to be needed for the best malformation markers.

DR. SKALKO: I'd like to ask Dr. Miller if he feels that since the epidemiological studies carried out in the past ten years have not, in fact revealed new human teratogens, if this effort is wasted as a diagnostic procedure?

DR. R. MILLER: I think it's been lost for that purpose by the time lag that has occurred. I think it has been valuable in other respects.

DR. LAWRENCE R. SHAPIRO (Letchworth Village, Thiells, New York): Dr. Miller implied that twins which are concordant for leukemia were assumed to be identical. Is any effort made to make this more than assumption, in view of the important data that can be obtained if we know for sure whether they are or not?

DR. R. MILLER: Our study was not the first to show the concordance rate for leukemia to be increased only in twins. The point is that, to date, every pair so described, and there are about twenty, have been of like sex, which I think would be unlikely if they were not identical. McMahon and Levy had five pairs, different from ours, in some of whom they were able to study zygosity. In each instance, the pairs were monozygous. Because of the confidentiality of the death certificates, we were unable to make the determination by tracing back.

DR. FLYNT: I'd like to comment on our surveillance program in Atlanta. We actually have looked at three specific episodes that we felt represented unusual occurrences. One was an apparent cluster of anencephaly that occurred at one hospital two summers ago. On further investigation we could find no identifiable relationship among the cases. A second one occurred last summer when we had a group of babies with tracheo-esophageal fistulae and four of them lived within an area about two miles in diameter in one county in Atlanta. Again, on interviewing these families, we were unable to find any relationship and, indeed, have found that clustering, based on the residence of children at birth is very untenable. In interviews with parents we found that 40% of them had changed residences between the time of conception and the time of birth. The third was in December of last year when there was a doubling in the incidence of children with

multiple malformations and, again, in interviewing parents we were unable to find any
association.

I would like to ask Dr. Miller if he is advo-
cating any particular method of surveillnace or
any particular technique for monitoring these
occurrences, or if he feels that several
approaches are feasible?

DR. R. MILLER: I am glad to hear about the
three specific episodes that you investigated.
I don't know if they have been recorded in the
monthly publications but it might be interesting
to do so.

EIS (Epidemic Intelligence Service) officers
have investigated congenital malformations.
There were two episodes of meningomyelocele, one
in Atlanta in the early 1960's, the other in
Jacksonville and although the number far exceeded
expectations in these areas, no causative factor
could be identified. I think the whole idea is
to use all possible modes of approach and not to
stick to just one.

EVALUATION OF VITAL RECORD USAGE FOR
CONGENITAL ANOMALY SURVEILLANCE

Philip Banister

Recognition of the thalidomide effect on the developing infant was a stunning blow to almost the whole medically sophisticated world. Subsequent difficulty in determining the number of infants who had been affected by this drug showed all too clearly the problems encountered in ascertaining the incidence of the various congenital anomalies.

Physicians, if one may generalize, have tended to be skeptical of the use of official records and documents -- surely this must have proved them right. Did no one ever look at the information available? This is rather a sobering thought -- after all the Bills of Mortality and Registers of Interment were passed in England in 1699. Following this, publications began to appear in the 18th and 19th centuries concerning the causes of infant death.[1,2]

It turns out that information on infants with thalidomide type deformities was recorded and changes in incidence of these anomalies were evident; unfortunately this information was not looked at until too late.[3] In the U.S.A. some workers had been making use of vital records for studies on congenital anomalies well before the thalidomide episode.[4] It appears then that the problem was not so much lack of information or lack of utilization but rather time of utilization.

With this brief introduction, I should like to discuss the evaluation of a program which uses vital records for monitoring the incidence of congenital anomalies in a defined population. I am indebted to Dr. J. Yerushalmy of the University of California, Berkeley.

The Reason for the Evaluation

For our purposes I think that we can assume that the primary reason is educational, we are gathered together to discuss the problem of surveillance and through this study hope to learn more about the value of this program and determine ways in which changes may be made to make future programs more effective.

The Description of the Program

I shall not go into the process which led to selection of documents, population, etc., but I shall describe how the program operated from January 1, 1966 until December 31, 1969 by the Child and Maternal Health Division, Department of National Health and Welfare, a modified program continues.

The population studied is really four populations consisting of the live and stillbirths occurring in New Brunswick, Manitoba, Alberta and British Columbia. The live births for these provinces for 1969 were: New Brunswick 11,863; Manitoba 18,267; Alberta 30,870; and British Columbia 35,515; a total of 96,515.

The documents used are the Physician's Notice of Birth, the medical section of the Stillbirth Registration form and the Death Certificate. The Physician's Notice of Birth is signed by the physician in attendance at the birth and must be completed within 24 or 48 hours after birth, depending on the province. Among the questions on the form is one concerning congenital anomalies. The Stillbirth form is completed for pregnancies of 20 weeks or more. The Death Certificate is referenced only for infants up to the age of one year.

The forms may be sent directly to the provincial registrar depending on the province, but so far as we are concerned no action is taken until they reach the central department. At this point they are screened for mention of a congenital anomaly by coding clerks, who do have access to a medical consultant. In practice we have asked that if there is any uncertainty the form is to be sent to us. If a provincial registry is using the same data these data may be sent first to the registry, the registry then forwarding them to Ottawa. The information is usually conveyed by photocopy of the original document; when it is transcribed, the exact wording of the original description is retained.

In Ottawa the documents are numbered individually. One clerk is responsible for this. The coding using I.C.D.A. codes is done by a pediatrician. The Research and Statistics Division of the Department is responsible for the preparation of punch cards on which is entered identifying information, date of birth and death, sex, I.C.D.A. code number. A card is made for each case, and one for each anomaly recorded. As further information is received the card is stamped "revise" and a new card is prepared to incorporate the fresh information. A surveillance table is prepared at one-two month intervals showing anomalies by the I.C.D.A. code, by province and by month of birth. This table is examined for trends and a copy is sent to the Provincial Department of Health. Should a suspicious trend develop then the actual contacting of physician and parents is done by the province. The key to success or failure of such a scheme rests with physician, who may or may not recognize and record a congenital anomaly. Lack of medical supervision is not a significant source of error, 99.3% of births occurred in hospitals in 1968. At the provincial level there is the possibility of a clerk not recognizing an anomaly recorded on one of the documents, and in Ottawa there may be failure to record and code an anomaly received from the province. Errors at the latter two levels are negligible, compared with those at the physician level.

Since this program was set up without an explicit statement of objective, we may assume that the ultimate objective is "to detect and eliminate from the environment of the developing embryo and fetus any teratogenic factor causing congenital anomalies" or in fact to reduce and eventually eliminate congenital anomalies.

Since neither of these objectives are measurable, we must set up more direct or immediate objectives as follows:

1. To record in the population under surveillance all congenital anomalies detectable in stillborn infants, and in live-born infants during the first year of life.
2. To establish baseline incidence rates for various anomalies or groups of anomalies.
3. To assess the significance of the recorded anomalies continuously or at frequent intervals.
4. To ensure follow-up of all cases associated with an increased incidence of anomalies.

While other objectives could be listed, for them to be of use for evaluation they must be measurable.

Working Assumptions

For the purpose of the evaluation we must assume that if all detectable congenital anomalies are recorded, and baseline incidence rates are established, and if the recorded anomalies are assessed frequently and all cases associated with an increased incidence of anomalies are followed up that we shall detect and eliminate teratogens.

Alternative Programs

These are programs which could also achieve the ultimate objective. We must compare our program with these alternates. Such programs are:

1. Retrieve and examine all embryos and fetuses from therapeutic and spontaneous abortions. Record all anomalies and establish baseline rates.

2. No program. The normal collection and publication of information shall continue. Detection of unusual events would depend upon the recognition by physicians of new syndromes. The congenital Rubella syndrome and thalidomide affected infants were delineated by this method.

This is an obvious place to comment very briefly on the two papers which were distributed in the pre-conference material, and which deal with the monitoring of the human population for mutagenesis.[5,6] While the need for detecting mutagens is undeniable, one must agree with Crow that the expense of any system of monitoring for mutagenesis could only be justified if it was also sensitive to teratogens.

Criteria

The baseline by which complete ascertainment of congenital anomalies is to be measured is impossible to state with certainty. Kennedy's[7] review of the world literature on the incidence

of congenital malformations yields a wide range
from less than 1% to more than 10% of newborns
affected. The average in the U.S.A., from
studies carried out using intensive examination,
is 8.8%. This contrasts strikingly with data
based upon official records, birth certificates
and retrospective questionnaires where only 0.8%
were reported, and hospital and clinic records
which recorded 1.3%. Following infants for a
longer period of time should increase the yield
and it would not be unreasonable to state that
8-10% of infants born after 20 weeks of pregnancy
and followed for a year might be expected to have
detectable anomalies. Arbitrarily, we shall de-
cide that if we record 4% of infants with anomalies we shall have achieved the objective. I am
deliberately avoiding dealing with the anomaly
rate since this is even more variable.

For the second objective, to establish baseline
rates for anomalies and groups of anomalies, we
shall select four groups of anomalies and compare
their incidence rates over four years of study.
If these rates do not fluctuate significantly
from year to year we shall have met our objective.

For the third objective, if we are able to
assess the recorded anomalies within two months
of birth or death in 75% of infants we shall have
met the objective.

For the fourth objective, the only situation in
which we have had to follow up cases has been
described elsewhere.[8] To achieve the objective
we shall need to have sufficient follow-up information to detect a recognized teratogen in 90% of
recorded cases.

Indices and Measures

I. To determine the proportion of infants with
recorded congenital anomalies up to the age of
one year we shall use the following ratio:

Number of infants with congenital anomalies recorded by Surveillance System up to first birthday
───
Provisional live births for the same population for the same period

II. To determine baseline rates for various anomalies and groups of anomalies. This objective will be measured by determining the incidence of anencephaly, spina bifida, cleft palate, lip, lip and palate and imperforate anus, for 1966-69 inclusive and assessing the variations between the four years. The overall rate for the four years will be compared with rates given by Stevenson and Källén.[9,10]

III. To measure the time interval between birth of an infant and assessment of an anomaly we shall assume that the date of mailing of information which is recorded on the punch card is within 2-3 days of coding and assessment. Using a table of random numbers we shall select 200 records from 1968 and 1969 and use the following ratio:

Number of cards in which information sent is 60 days or less later than birth date of infant
───
Number of cards selected using table of random numbers

To measure follow-up cases we shall use the following ratio:

Number of completed follow-up reports received for infants with congenital reduction deformities of limbs
───
Number of infants with congenital reduction deformities of limbs known to surveillance system and born in 1969

Evaluation Design

To allow comparison of our program with an alternate we shall select another province not participating in the scheme. The population of this province is rather similar to the total population of the four provinces in our program and not dissimilar in terms of infant mortality rate.

The alternate program operates using the same three forms as in our program, these being forwarded to the provincial registrar and copies going to those concerned with maternal and child health. While the forms may be glanced at, no tabulations are made. Some two years later a special report is issued from which incidence rates for congenital anomalies are available.

Follow-up of infants with reduction deformities was done at our request and was by means of a letter sent directly to the physician who had signed the form reporting the anomaly.

The actual analysis then will be done by:

a) Evaluation of our program on the basis of whether or not the four immediate objectives were achieved.

b) A comparison with the achievements of the alternate program.

c) A rough estimate of the achievements of the program in terms of cost/benefit.

Measures for objective one.

	Ratio	Percent	Criterion
Program	$\dfrac{5737}{376,481} \times 100$	1.5	4%
Alternate	$\dfrac{7350}{553,790} \times 100$	1.3	4%

For objective two, Tables I and II and Figure I give some figures for the number of anomalies by year for our program and the alternate program. It may be seen that for these anomalies anyway, there is little fluctuation, and certainly no statistically significant fluctuation. The same is true for the alternate program. Data from two other studies are shown.

Objectives three and four.

		Program	Criterion
Number of cases assessed within 60 days of birth	171 x 100	85.5%	75%
Number of records sampled	200		

Alternate program: no information is available.

Objective four, 45 infants with congenital deformities of the limbs born in 1969 were reported to us.

			Criterion
Follow up	$\frac{37}{45}$	= 82%	90%
Alternate program	$\frac{14}{24*}$	= 58%	90%

*Born January-June 1969

Analysis and Conclusions
    Using the arbitrary rules set up for our evaluation we have reached two of our four objectives. In one of these, the ongoing surveillance of anomalies, there is a clearcut difference between our program and the alternate. Because only 1.5% of infants are notified as having congenital anomalies compared with our objective of 4%, fluctuations in reporting might easily obscure

changes in incidence. It is well known that an article in a medical journal can influence the proportion of cases reported. One of the most important steps in evaluation which we have not been able to take is a verification of the accuracy of reporting, but from follow-up of those infants with reduction deformities of the limbs, out of 45 cases born in 1969 known from all sources, 42 were reported to our surveillance system and were verified. There were actually 48 cases, three were discarded because of inaccurate diagnosis.

To return to the question of ascertainment, another approach to evaluation of this might be to select an anomaly or group of anomalies and then try to discover how many infants had this anomaly in the population. In British Columbia the registry for Handicapped Children and Adults accepts notification from many sources and at any age. With the kind cooperation of Dr. James Miller, Mr. John Doughty and Miss Anne Scott, we are starting to compare our cases with theirs, but have not yet completed these studies.

Part of our evaluation should compare the cost to benefit ratio of our program and the alternate program. Until such time as the program detects and eliminates a teratogen this is not possible. We can, however, give a rough estimate of the cost to yield ratio. This program is cheap because it utilizes information already being collected for other purposes, costs are confined to staff, stationery and postage, plus some processing charges.

While I have a breakdown of how the total cost of $33,828.50 was arrived at, I do not believe the details are of interest to this group.

From the estimated cost of the program we arrived at a figure of:

$ .35 per birth monitored

$16.38 per anomaly recorded
$23.07 per case recorded.

Unfortunately, it was not possible to obtain a value for the cost of the alternate program.

It will become apparent later that the yield has been considerably increased by the changes in the program I shall describe, so that although the cost of monitoring each birth remains the same, it now costs $5.78 per anomaly and $8.18 per case recorded.

I should like briefly to describe the changes made to improve this program. For some years a federally supported Hospital Insurance program has been in effect. This requires the completion of a record for each individual born in, or admitted to hospitals. Since the start of 1970, we have been including information derived from this source in our study. As might be expected this has led to an increased yield of cases and anomalies. A study was done last year using 1968 data and if we recalculate the index used earlier to give the yield of cases for two provinces for 1968 we get the following results:

P.N.O.B. Stillbirths Deaths)	Cases Births	$\dfrac{387}{29,031}$	=	1.3%
Hospital Insurance Records	Cases Births	$\dfrac{883}{29,031}$	=	3.0%
Combined Records (no duplicates)	Cases	$\dfrac{1,092}{29,031}$	=	3.8%

or pretty close to our criterion of 4% for achieving the first objective.

In conclusion, I have presented an approach to evaluation of a surveillance system set up to monitor the incidence of congenital anomalies in infants by using existing sources of information. We have measured the achievements of this program indirectly with a liberal use of working assumptions, and have compared these achievements with an existing method of vital statistics collection. Some changes in the program made as a result of our experience have been described and I have concluded that such a program may provide useful information about the incidence of congenital anomalies for a very modest expenditure. The final proof of such a program must remain the detection of a teratogen.

ACKNOWLEDGEMENTS

Members of the Biostatistics Division of the Research and Statistics Directorate, Department of National Health and Welfare, prepared data for evaluation and performed the statistical analyses. This study could not have been carried out without the unfailing cooperation of colleagues in New Brunswick, Manitoba, Alberta and British Columbia. Mrs. Yoneko Kawamoto, Division of Child and Maternal Health, prepared the tables and figures.

REFERENCES

1. Ballexserd, J.: Dissertation sur cette question: Quelles sont les cause principales de la mort d'un aussi grand nombres d'enfants, et quels sont les preservatifs les plus efficaces et les plus simples pour leur conserver la vie? Genève, 1775.
2. Watt, Robert: Treatise on the History, Nature and Treatment of Chincough, 1813.
3. Leck, I., Smithells, R.W.: The ascertainment of malformations. Lancet 1:101-103, 1963.

4. DePorte, J.V., Parkhurst, E: Congenital malformations and birth injuries among children born in New York State, outside of New York City, in 1940-1942. New York State J. Med. 45:1097, 1945.
5. National Institute of Environmental Health Sciences, National Institutes of Health, U.S. Public Health Service: Report of the Committee for the Study of Monitoring of Human Mutagenesis.
6. Crow, James F.: Human Population Monitoring. Paper number 1362 from the Genetics Laboratory, University of Wisconsin, Madison.
7. Kennedy, W.P.: Epidemiologic Aspects of the Problem of Congenital Malformations. Birth Defects. Original Article Series, Vol. III: No.2, December,1967.
8. Banister, Philip: Congenital malformations: preliminary report of an investigation of reduction deformities of the limbs, triggered by a pilot surveillance system. Can. Med. Assoc. J. 103: 466-472, 1970.
9. Stevenson, Alan C., Johnston, Harold A., Stewart, M.I. Patricia, et al.: Congenital Malformations, A Report of a Study of Series of Consecutive Births in 24 Centres. Supplement to Vol. 34 Bulletin of the World Health Organization, 1966.
10. Källén, Bengt, Winberg, Jan: A Swedish Register of Congenital Malformations: Experience with continuous registration during 2 years with special reference to multiple malformations. Pediatrics 41:765-783, 1968.

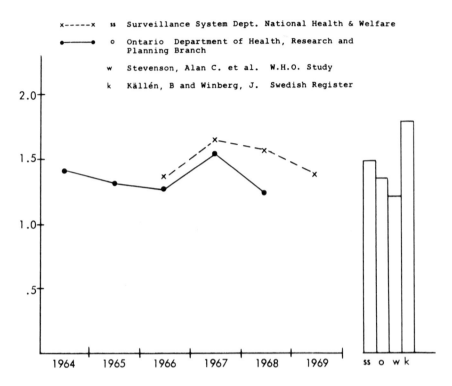

Figure 1. Cleft lip, cleft palate, cleft lip and palate. Various studies.

BIRTH DEFECTS MONITORING

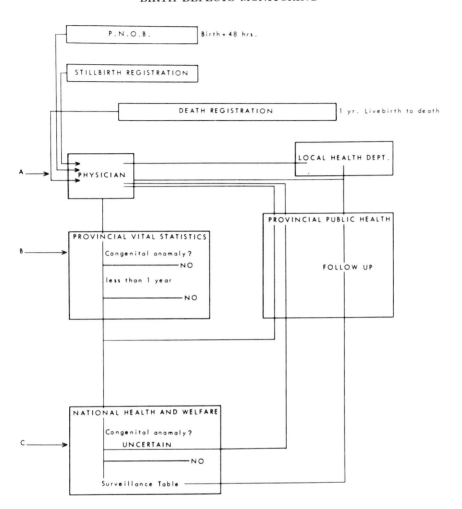

Figure 2. Surveillance System.

Table 1

INCIDENCE RATES SELECTED ANOMALIES

ANOMALY	1966		1967		1968		1969		TOTAL	
	Cases	Rate[1]	Cases	Rate[1]	Cases	Rate[1]	Cases	Rate[1]	Cases	Rate[1]
Anencephaly	69	.74	73	.78	77	.83	70	.73	289	.77
Spina bifida	127	1.35	112	1.20	114	1.23	105	1.09	458	1.22
Cleft lip Cleft palate Cleft lip & palate	127	1.35	154	1.65	147	1.58	135	1.40	563	1.50
Imperforate anus	22	.23	26	.28	22	.24	25	.26	95	.25
BIRTHS	93,823		93,276		92,867		96,515		376,481	

1. Per 1,000 births.
2. Department of Nutritional Health and Welfare.

134

Table 2

INCIDENCE RATES SELECTED ANOMALIES

VARIOUS STUDIES

ANOMALY	TOTAL		ONTARIO		STEVENSON		KALLEN	
	Cases	Rate[1]	Cases	Rate[1]	Cases	Rate[1]	Cases	Rate[1]
Anencephaly	289	.77	559*	1.01	436	1.05	-	.37
Spina bifida	458	1.22	776	1.40	399	.96	-	1.09
Cleft lip Cleft palate Cleft lip and palate	563	1.50	765	1.38	504	1.21	-	1.79
Imperforate anus	95	.25	-	-	72	.17	-	.29
BIRTHS	376,481		553,790		416,695		159,500	

1. Per 1,000 births.
* ICD Code 750 Monstrosity including Anencephaly.

135

EXPERIENCE WITH MALFORMATION SURVEILLANCE

Samuel Milham, Jr.

In May, 1962, I started a malformation surveillance system, using the birth and still birth
records filed in Upstate New York as a source of
cases. The sole purpose of the system was to
detect as soon as possible any unusual incidence
of birth malformations. I ran the system until
December, 1966. Since November, 1967, I have
operated a similar system at the Washington State
Health Department. The details of setting up and
operating the New York system have been published
previously.[1] The system simply counts reported
malformations by type, county of birth and month
of birth. It compares the current monthly experience to the experience developed over previous
time periods. This presentation will be devoted
to a brief discussion of experience with the
system.

In both New York and Washington, a small number
of quirks or artifacts in malformation reporting
have come to light. For example, one New York
physician reports nearly all his male deliveries
as having "congenital phimosis". This was
noticed quickly, since the rural county where he
practiced had as many cases in the miscellaneous
genito-urinary rubric as did the rest of the
state. A similar reporting artifact was noted in

Washington records. A physician on a large obstetric service reports an extraordinary frequency of minor malformations (nevi, hydrocele, and undescended testicle) with no corresponding increase of major malformations. Malformation frequencies and rates for his county are therefore adjusted for the rubrics which are systematically over-reported. Initially a number of case reports were followed up before deciding that this "epidemic" was due to overzealous reporting. This experience suggests that the reporting physician should be an analytic variable in malformation incidence studies which use physicians' reports, and that appropriate denominators should be developed.

The surveillance system has had two tests in the course of its operation: a rubella epidemic and what I believe was a "mini-epidemic" of phocomelia due to thalidomide.

Details of the surveillance system were worked out before the thalidomide incident was known. Baseline data for malformation expectation was obtained in the course of retrospective studies[2,3] using the New York vital record file. Fortunately, the malformation code used for these studies and for surveillance had a specific rubric for reduction deformities of the arms and/or legs. The first 8 months of operation of the New York system saw phocomelia cases reported at over twice the expected frequency, based on 10 years experience, 1950-1960 (see Table I). Evidence that this increase was due to thalidomide is provided by the fact that thalidomide was mentioned on the birth records of 2 cases, after the European experience became public, by the timing of the increase, and by the nature of the reported malformations. Table I also shows that reduction deformity frequency returned to expected levels in 1963, giving support to the hypothesis that the increase in cases was due to thalidomide.

A second test of the system came in 1964, when New York state suffered an epidemic of rubella. Reported rubella peaked in April, 1964, with 11,266 reported cases (see Table 2). Since reported cases make up only a small fraction of all cases, (probably less than 5%) there can be no question that a sizable number of pregnant women and fetuses were exposed to the virus during the epidemic. The total teratogenic impact of the epidemic, as measured by the surveillance system, was small, but the system did detect an increase in reported eye malformations, including cataract, 8 to 9 months after the rubella peak (see Table 2). The fetal death rate and total malformation rate also hit maxima for the study period, 8 to 9 months after the rubella peak. No marked trend in total live births was discernable, although births in November and December, 1964, were low for the year. Births in January-February, 1965, were also lower than in the same period in 1964. This was a period, however, of a general decline in the birth rate. To keep things in perspective, even in an epidemic, rubella can only account for a small proportion of reported malformations.

Changes in the surveillance system have been few. I added a code rubric for microtia in anticipation of the rubella episode. Also, a rubric for the various chromosomal syndromes has been added.

Initially, I graphed the malformation frequencies each month but now simply make a frequency table of malformations by type by month of birth, and by type by county by month of birth.

In the eight years during which the system has been operating, no unexplained "epidemic" of malformations has come to my attention. Admittedly, vital records are crude and incomplete

sources of malformation information. I am con-
vinced, however, that an epidemic of malformations obvious at birth will be detected by such
a system, since the entire live born and still
born population of the state is under surveillance. The New York phocomelia and rubella experience support this conviction.

REFERENCES

1. Milham, S.: Congenital malformation surveillance system based on vital records. Public
Health Reports 78:448-452, 1963.
2. Gittelsohn, A.M., Milham, S.: Vital record
incidence of congenital malformations in New York
State. Public Service Publication No. 1163: 305-
314, 1965.
3. Gittelsohn, A.M., Milham, S.: Declining Incidence of central nervous system anomalies in
New York State. British J. of Prev. and Soc.
Med. 16: 153-158, 1962.

Table 1

Frequency of absence of arms or legs or parts
thereof, except digits by 8 month period
May, 1962 - August, 1965

Upstate New York birth and stilbirth records

Time	Cases	
	Expected*	Observed
May, 1962 - December, 1962	8	19
January, 1963 - August, 1963	8	8
September, 1963 - April, 1964	8	9
May, 1964 - December, 1964	8	7
January, 1965 - August, 1965	8	8

*1950 - 1960 experience averaged 12 cases per
year

Table 2

Reported Rubella Cases, Fetal Death Rate, Malformation Rate, Frequency of Cataract plus Eye Malformation and Live Births Reported on Birth and Stillbirth Records, Upstate New York, December, 1963 - May, 1965

Year	Month	Rubella Cases Reported	Fetal Death Rate per 10,000 total Births	Malformation Rate per 10,000 total Births	Cataract and/or Eye Malformations	Live Births
1963	December	264	150.9	105.3	1	15,572
1964	January	1,202	133.8	113.7	1	15,467
	February	3,855	138.0	118.7	2	15,406
	March	8,997	140.2	114.7	4	16,038
	April	11,266	150.0	109.6	3	15,594
	May	8,211	129.8	118.7	0	16,249
	June	4,940	150.8	119.5	2	16,307
	July	1,258	148.4	110.3	3	17,313
	August	315	144.8	122.9	1	16,436
	September	85	168.7	123.5	2	16,473
	October	47	142.6	106.9	1	16,546
	November	110	158.7	119.4	3	14,991
	December	46	171.3	123.9	11	15,406
1965	January	**	155.9	135.6	6	14,815
	February	**	145.1	109.7	2	13,845
	March	**	147.2	117.8	2	15,617
	April	**	151.9	105.5	1	14,871
	May	**	151.6	107.3	1	15,561

FEASIBILITY OF VITAL AND HOSPITAL RECORD
LINKAGE IN MONITORING BIRTH DEFECTS

Alan M. Gittelsohn

One aspect of monitoring carries with it an implication of population surveillance and the organization of broadly based systems of observation whereby the incidence of birth defects can be measured in a spatial and temporal context. Presumably, the occurrence of a detectable increase over time or of a geographical clustering of cases would be the signal for the initiation of investigations directed at identification of underlying causes. From a population standpoint, a further implication is that such data systems increase the possibility of early detection of shifts in incidence. While these propositions remain to be tested and demonstrated by concrete experience, it is largely because relatively little work has been done in the area and few opportunities to do so have arisen. As contrasted with reliance on individual observation, informal communication mechanisms and ad hoc investigation, justification for the introduction of monitoring systems necessarily must rely on extrapolation from prior instances of successful detection. In terms of the examples of phocomelia, congenital cataract and retrolental fibroplasia, it is a moot point whether, before the fact, we would have been able to design a method for monitoring with the capability of signaling the unusual occurrence of these conditions or, even if present in the data, would have been noted by the data analyzers.

A monitoring system, to be of use, must be able to detect an unambiguous and rapid response to the introduction of a new teratogenic agent through study of both the recognized cases and the population from which the cases are derived. To this end, the design and development of new approaches to monitoring must be weighed against modification and enhancement of methods currently available for surveillance. At the present, vital records constitute the only centrally organized data system in the country which has attained complete population coverage. Uses and limitations of the birth record for monitoring congenital defects have been noted by prior speakers. Generally, the birth certificate is filed too early for all but the gross external defects and defects incompatible with extended post-natal survival to be detected and recorded. Wide variability exists between institutions in diagnostic standards, diagnostic acumen and the degree of assiduousness with which data are recorded. Despite the problems of completeness and comparability, the birth record possesses a potential as an underlying building block in a data system whereby information from diverse medical and health record sources is collated into a single patient history.

Present focus will be on such potentialities and on the problems of extending the information content of vital records through computerized linkage with hospital records. The underlying assumption is that there is value in assembling existing health data pertaining to a single individual as long as the cost remains modest. The increasing range and decreasing costs of digital computers, together with the current development of making accessible files of hospital data open the possibility of assembling individual case histories on a routine and massive scale. Experience in several linkage projects have demonstrated cost feasibility and, in fact, additional savings might accrue if the same linked files were available to different users who previously maintained their own data independently.

The experience on which this discussion is based relates to an on-going study of the population of the State of Vermont being carried out by the Northern New England Regional Medical Program. Records of natality, mortality, morbidity and hospitalization are being collected for the entire state in the development of an information base for characterizing aspects of the medical care system. Since the work has been initiated only recently, the remarks will be restricted to approaches rather than results.

Hospital record systems

The past decade has been witness to a rapid growth throughout the United States of computerized hospital discharge abstract systems containing diagnostic data of direct relevance to monitoring. Specific pressures for hospital inpatient information of various types have spurred this development at an increasing pace to the point where all of the hospitalizations in certain states and in regions of other states are included in particular discharge abstracting programs. The primary motivation for the generation of hospital information is not the provision of data for studies of incidence or for epidemiological research, but is couched in such terms as "utilization review", "medical audit" and "hospital management". For the latter purposes, the type of information collected emphasizes procedures and services provided. Nevertheless, the hospital discharge abstract systems

have led to the creation of extensive data files
which may lend themselves as input to methodologies for the surveillance of certain types of
birth defects.

A number of distinctive and sometimes competing
and overlapping programs have evolved at national,
regional and local levels under voluntary hospital participation. The largest of the hospital
data systems, the Professional Activities Study
(PAS) of the Commission of Professional and
Hospital Activities, reported in 1969 the participation of over 1,300 hospitals representing
30 percent of all short-term general hospitalizations in the United States and Canada. In a
few states and in several metropolitan areas
almost total coverage has been attained. Other
hospital abstracting systems, with the primary
purpose of providing services to hospitals, oper-
ate within states under the aegis of medical and
hospital associations. While types of information collected are individualistic and not
standardized, a common core consists of minimal
demographic items, particulars pertaining to the
hospital episode and as many as eight coded
diagnoses.

Incidence studies based on information ascertained as a result of hospitalization present
major and sometimes insurmountable problems.
Particular hospital samples tend to be biased,
non-representative and heterogeneous in that admission to a specific facility may be dictated by
a series of extraneous factors. While pooling of
information for all hospitals in a given area may
overcome this type of difficulty, it poses the
additional problem of data comparability. There
is little standardization among physicians in the
collection and recording of patient data and
there are few uniformly applied criteria for de-
fining and classifying patient history, physical

findings and diagnoses. Weed,[1] a profound
student of medical records, describes what he
terms a remarkable spectrum of behavior among
practicing physicians in establishing the
patient's data base ranging from the compulsively
elaborate to the chronically haphazard. He
characterizes current practices of observing and
recording medical data along the lines of a "game
of football with a random number of players on a
field of no definite length." At the least, it
can be said that any monitoring system based on
records collected from different institutions
will be subject to important limitations in this
regard.

Retrieval and record linkage

It has long been recognized that a wide range
of information pertaining to a single individual
is stored throughout diverse and independent
record systems. The desirability of collating
routine data into a single file has been considered in a number of different contexts and a
few years ago gave rise to advocacy of the establishment of "data banks" to be used for a variety
of purposes. Developments in the computer field,
including the increasingly rapid input and output
devices and the growing sizes and decreasing
access time of immediate memories, have made all
types of record linkage projects economically
feasible. Pioneering work in the linkage and
collation of medical records by Newcombe[2] in
Canada and by the Oxford Group in England[3] has
stirred much interest and commentary but relatively little in the way of direct applications in
the United States.

A major difficulty with all medical linkage of
efforts has been the lack of a universal and
unique patient identifier whereby an individual
could be traced through his contacts with

different components of the medical care system. To avoid problems of confidentiality of records and to insure wide participation, most hospital discharge abstracting systems have restricted patient identification to a bare minimum of demographic items such as sex and age. The result is that the unit of observation is an episode of hospitalization which cannot be related readily to readmissions of the same patient. Advocacy of unique person identification by assignment of a social security number at birth or a birth number based on encoding of name, date and other characteristics has received little favorable response. In fact, active opposition seems to be the current political climate. While a National Health Service number is issued at birth in the United Kingdom, apparently it has not proved acceptable to require this number on hospital records. Since uniqueness is not attainable, attention has centered on the possibility of linking records on the basis of non-unique identifiers and characteristics, any one of which, taken separately, may be insufficient to provide definitive evidence for or against the match of a given pair of records, but which taken collectively may serve the purpose quite effectively.

In record linkage applications, since no unique identifier is generally available, matching is carried out under uncertainty, using a set of attributes common to the files. Even with files of modest size, it is necessary to restrict searching to subsets defined on the basis of variables of a "rule-out" type which impose the requirement for exact agreement. The latter are selected on the basis of discriminating power, constancy over time and low noise level. Examples might include sex, origin and birthdate. A second type of attribute used on a "rule-in" basis includes those variables, fortuitously carried in the files to be linked, which may provide evidence for but not against a match of a particular record pair. Any odd bit and piece of information with some power of discrimination such as patient's address, diagnoses, weight or attending physician, all of which are subject to change over time, may be used for this purpose.

A linkage procedure is a search strategy and a set of rules for determining when a pair of records constitutes a match. The success of such a procedure is related to its cost-utility, specificity and sensitivity. While measures for the latter can easily be constructed in terms of the number of correct matches, (true positives) incorrect matches, (false positives) and missed matches, (false negatives) only the cost side of cost-utility is subject to direct measurement and then only within the confines of a specific strategy. The speed and accuracy of record matching depends on the structure imposed on the files to be linked. Several different kinds of file organization are described in the information retrieval literature, including such methods as batching, key transformation, chaining and table hierarchy. Of particular note are the so-called "optimal" single and multistage systems based on combinatorial analysis and projective geometry of Ray-Chaudhuri.[4] It is not the purpose here to review the various alternatives in any detail but merely to note that even simple, inefficient approaches result in tolerable cost levels when utilizing high speed, large memory computers.

Study of Vermont records

Types of linked files involving various degrees of complexity are being studied. The simplest form, which involves no more than standard data processing techniques, relates to the hospitalizations of patients within a single institution maintaining a unit numbering system. Greater difficulties are encountered with the extension of patient histories to include linkages between records of different hospitals in the state. The problem in formulating an approach is that there is little basis for estimating the number of multiplicities to be expected for a single patient or the time lapse between admissions. Inter-hospital matching is of importance for children with several types of birth defects initially admitted to a community hospital and subsequently referred to more specialized facilities. Many conditions involving surgical intervention are in this category. Other types of linkages include birth with death records and both birth and death records with hospital abstracts. Because different sets of identifiers are available for the various types of linkage applications, a separate approach is required for each type.

In a simple example of matching birth records of Vermont residents and discharge abstracts within hospitals, a reasonably high degree of accuracy was obtained with only four identifying variables -- sex, birthdate, residence and birth weight measured in ounces. Other than the slippage in out-of-state hospital use occurring at the borders, the major cause of missed matches was clerical and key punching errors. Because of asymmetries in weight, the approach was sensitive enough to correctly distinguish the records of most like-sexed twins who in other respects share the same characteristics.

Preliminary results of assembling single case histories from vital records and hospital records of children under two years of age for 1968 and 1969 are unsurprising. Birth certificate recording of congenital anomalies is evidently

highly variable, depending primarily on identification of the defect by external examination.
The combined vital record incidence of all malformations of about 1.3 percent in the particular
birth cohort was increased by over two and one-
half fold when hospital information was added to
the data file. In part, the difference was due
to failure to record information on the birth
certificate when the defect was observable at
birth and, in part, due to ascertainment of cases
after the immediate perinatal period. The latter
was particularly important for heart defects
compatible with post-natal survival, for congenital pyloric stenosis and for other defects of
internal organs.

Since the linked file is based on a total birth
cohort together with all records of hospitalizations contained in the system, irrespective of
diagnosis, the assembled data provides for the
possibility of investigating a number of conditions and outcomes which may be related to
events occurring in the perinatal period. Of
relevance to monitoring in this respect are the
childhood cancers and leukemia. While Vermont,
with fewer than 10,000 births per year, is too
small to provide sufficient case material for
detailed studies of specific defects and disease
entities, extension of the methodology to other
areas is direct.

CONCLUSION

The organization of efficient monitoring
systems for detecting changes in the incidence of
birth defects requires specificity of classification, complete and early recognition of cases
as they occur and improvement of methods for the
collection and dissemination of data concerning
potentially important conditions. The possibil-

ity of utilizing existing vital record and hospital record systems to fulfill these requirements warrants further exploration. The development of computer methodologies for record linkage and the rapid growth of automated hospital discharge abstracting systems has made such work possible. It is now clear that linkage can be carried out with a high degree of reliability if sufficient numbers of attributes and characteristics are included in the records without using names or resorting to unique person identification schemes and thereby avoiding the maintaining of confidentiality of records. Newcombe[5] asserts that the unit cost of linking an incoming record is about one mil. While somewhat lower than that achieved in our own experience, the total cost of an on-going linkage system should be modest since the amount of resources available for monitoring will not be great. In contrast with organizing and promoting notification systems solely for congenital defects, computer linkage of birth, death and hospital records offers the possibility of developing more complete data at a reasonable price.

REFERENCES

1. Weed, L.L.: Medical Records, Medical Education and Patient Care. The Press of Case Western Reserve University, Cleveland, 1969.
2. Newcombe, H.B.: Record linking: the design of efficient systems for linking records into individual and family histories. Amer. J. Hum. Genet. 19:335-348, 1967
3. Acheson, E.D., (Ed.): Record Linkage in Medicine. Edinburgh, E. and S. Livingstone Ltd., 1968.
4. Ray-Chaudhure, D.K.: Combinatorial information retrieval systems for files. SIAM J.

Appl. Math. 16:973-992, 1968.
5. Newcombe, H.B.: Value of Canadian Hospital
Insurance records in detecting increases in congenital anomalies. Canad. Med. Assn. J. 101:
121-128, 1969.

METROPOLITAN ATLANTA CONGENITAL DEFECTS PROGRAM

J. William Flynt, Jr.[1]
Allan J. Ebbin [1]
Godfrey P. Oakley, Jr.[1]
Arthur Falek[2]
Clark W. Heath, Jr.[1]

The Metropolitan Atlanta Congenital Defects Program is a joint project begun in October 1967 by the Division of Human Genetics, Georgia Mental Health Institute, the Departments of Psychiatry, Obstetrics and Gynecology and Pediatrics, Emory University School of Medicine and the Center for Disease Control.

Its purpose is to conduct surveillance of malformations in a metropolitan area containing a registry for use in epidemiologic and genetic studies of congenital malformations. From our experience, we feel that such a registry can be used for other purposes as well. For instance, state and local health departments should consider malformation surveillance and registries as a way to identify more quickly infants and families with malformations in need of medical,

---

[1]Congenital Malformations Unit and Leukemia Section, C.D.C.

[2]Division of Medical Genetics, Georgia Mental Health Institute.

nursing, or financial assistance.

For surveillance purposes our definition of a "malformation" includes any structural, chromosomal or biochemical abnormality in an infant diagnosed before his first birthday. However, care is taken to distinguish infants whose malformations are diagnosed at less than 7 days of age, since detection and reporting of malformations in this group are more reliable and complete than for older infants.

The surveillance program encompasses a five-county metropolitan area with a population of 1.3 million by the 1970 census, with approximately 26,000 births annually. Seventy-seven percent of the population is white; the other 23 percent is predominantly Negro. There are 21 hospitals, one of which is limited to pediatrics.

Infants with malformations are registered primarily through visits by one of the surveillance staff to hospital nurseries, delivery rooms, and medical record departments. These visits vary from twice a week at the largest to monthly at the smaller hospital. Nursing personnel in the hospitals provide names of infants with malformations. In some they enter the name of an infant with a malformation in a book provided by us, while in others we depend upon the nurses to remember the infants and malformations. This data is supplemented by copies of stillbirth and infant death certificates furnished by the Georgia Health Department. Other sources for registering cases include the four chromosome laboratories of the city, pathology reports of the two largest hospitals and cases reported by practicing physicians coincidental to requests for consultations or for information on malformations.

An integral part of surveillance is to return

the data in an analyzed form to the people who
provide it. We do this through a monthly report
which monitors individual malformations by
giving the number of cases that have occurred
that month within the metropolitan area by
county and by month of birth. These cases are
compared with the number occurring in preceding
months and years. Whenever a significant increase in cases is noted, the families of the
infants involved are interviewed concerning
possible environmental exposures. Since the
inception of surveillance three such "case
clusters" have been noted and investigated. In
none was an explanation found for the increase
in incidence or the clustering of cases.

A number of people work on the surveillance
program. A nurse, whose salary is paid by the
Georgia Mental Health Institute, a physician
epidemiologist, and an experienced interviewer
conduct surveillance and interview mothers deliv-
ering infants with selected malformations. In
addition, there are clerical, statistical and
secretarial staff who work on other CDC projects,
but also devote time to malformation surveillance.
For data analysis we use the computer system and
programming staff at the Center for Disease
Control.

Fifty thousand dollars is a reasonable estimate
of the annual cost of conducting surveillance and
processing the Atlanta data. This figure covers
the related expenses of the collaborating institutions but it does not cover the cost of studies
conducted in addition to surveillance. The use
of less highly trained individuals in gathering
the data would lower the cost. From our experience this substitution could probably be done
once a smoothly-functioning reporting system is
underway and hospital personnel are accustomed to

surveillance. On the other hand, we have found that the nurse and physician have been of assistance in confirming diagnoses, recommending facilities for care and increasing the awareness of malformations in the medical and nursing communities. This is one of the subtle but important ancillary benefits of a program of this type within a community.

FETAL SEQUELAE OF RUBELLA IMMUNIZATION AND BIRTH DEFECTS PROGRAM IN LOS ANGELES COUNTY*

Allan J. Ebbin
Miriam G. Wilson

Pregnancy is a contraindication for rubella vaccination since it is not known whether the rubella vaccine, which is live, although attenuated virus, can damage the fetus when given to a pregnant woman. Even though the vaccine is not recommended for women of reproductive age, it seemed likely that some women unaware of their pregnancy, would be vaccinated. The assessment of the fetal risk from rubella vaccine is the main objective of our study.

In July of 1969 we began a surveillance program of congenital rubella and possible sequelae of rubella immunization in Los Angeles County. Information about the possible embryopathic effect of rubella vaccine is being sought by two methods: 1) prospective clinical and virus laboratory studies of pregnancies where vaccine has been administered; and 2) surveillance of birth defects and illness in newly born infants for evidence of fetal rubella infection, and subse-

---

*This study is supported by the National Center for Disease Control -- Grant Number 1R01CC00482-01.

sequent investigation of pregnancy history. Appropriate control pregnancies and births are studied for comparison. Area physicians, three county hospitals, five private hospitals, the Los Angeles County Health Department and the Los Angeles County Unified School Districts are cooperating in this investigation.

Public Health nurses visit the participating hospitals at least three times each week and interview all mothers who have answered affirmatively to the admission questionnaire regarding rubella immunization, contact or disease. A precoded answer form is used in these interviews. The nurses also ascertain whether any infants have been born with malformations or with neonatal illness suggesting rubella infection. Pediatricians, obstetricians, and general practitioners of Los Angeles County, contacted through letters and at hospital medical staff meetings, are requested to refer women who have received the vaccine during or shortly before pregnancy or who have had a household contact with a vaccine recipient during that time period.

For each study patient a control patient is selected on the basis of matched maternal age, race and parity, family socio-economic status, and sex of infant. Complete clinical and laboratory data are obtained for control and study patients.

When a maternal history discloses rubella vaccine or rubella infection, hemagglutination inhibition (HI) antibody titers and throat and rectal swabs for virus isolation are obtained from the mother and the infant. When spontaneous or therapeutic abortion occurs, abortus tissue is obtained for viral isolation.

Twenty-three women who received rubella vaccine shortly before or early in pregnancy are currently being studied. The time of vaccination ranges from 84 days before to about 88 days after

the last menstrual period. Most of these women
were not evaluated by pre-vaccine HI titers.
Most of these women were not on a reliable contra-
ceptive program at the time they were vaccinated.*
Approximately one-third of the mothers have
delivered apparently normal infants, who are
being followed for at least two years. The other
women have had spontaneous or therapeutic
abortions or are still pregnant. The therapeutic
abortions were obtained for maternal mental
health indications because of the possibility of
a severely malformed child resulting from the
vaccine.

In the first year of our study 155 infants with
congenital defects have been reported from the
participating hospitals, representing an incidence of major birth defects of 8.2 per 1,000
(155/18,862 live births). The incidence of
birth defects found in this study is less than
that found in most newborn surveys. An even
higher incidence has been found in those surveys
where infants are followed for longer periods of
time or those which include genetic, metabolic or
molecular disorders and minor malformations. An
analysis of drug usage during pregnancy, maternal
disease and parental ages in the study group compared with the control group is planned for a
later time when adequate numbers are available
for study.

Twelve infants were found to have congenital
rubella syndrome, all resulting from natural
rubella infection of the mother during pregnancy.
Five of these infants were referred to the Los

---

*Chin, J., Ebbin, A.J., Wilson, M.G. and Lennette,
E.H., Avoidance of rubella immunization of women
during or shortly before pregnancy. J. A. M. A.
In press, 1970.

Angeles County-USC Medical Center from outside hospitals not directly participating in this program. Rubella virus was isolated from the throat and/or rectal swab from nine of these infants. Twelve infants with congenital rubella syndrome represent a large number for a non-rubella epidemic year in Los Angeles County, particularly since complete ascertainment is unlikely even by this study. For 1969-1970, we estimate that Los Angeles County had about 0.37 cases per 1,000 live births or one in 2,700 live births.*

At this time we do not know whether rubella vaccine has embryopathic effects, since an insufficient number of pregnancies at risk have been studied. We do not know whether the mothers who were not tested before vaccination for presence of rubella antibody were at risk; they may have been immune. Furthermore, it is possible that the rubella vaccine has a low teratogenic effect. Under these circumstances it is necessary to study a large number of non-immune women who receive the vaccine at a critical time in pregnancy before the teratogenic safety of this vaccine can be determined.

ACKNOWLEDGEMENT

The following hospitals are participating in this study: Children's Hospital of Los Angeles, the Hospital of the Good Samaritan Medical Center, Harbor General Hospital, Hollywood Presbyterian Hospital, Huntington Memorial Hospital, John Wesley Hospital, Los Angeles County-USC Medical Center, St. John's Hospital and White

---

* Incidence based on cases/known total number of births from which cases were derived.

Memorial Hospital. Miss Irene Olsakowski, PHN, Mrs. Eileen Newton, PHN and Mrs. Carol Nicholson, PHN, assisted in data and sample collection. Viral studies are being performed at the Infectious Disease Laboratory, University of Southern California, School of Medicine. The Los Angeles County Health Department and the Los Angeles City Unified School Districts assisted in detection of cases.

DISCUSSION

DR. R. MILLER: I would like to make one comment. It seems that one of the features of today's presentation has been that any system that works can be tested, perhaps, with regard to rubella syndrome occurrence. I was particularly impressed with Dr. Milham's demonstration that his system works in its ability to detect the effects of rubella, despite some of the incompleteness that must exist in the reporting. Dr. Ebbin also suggested that rubella syndrome can be can be used to test his system. The NINDS studies, as I mentioned this morning, didn't work, suggesting that that approach is not the most effective one and that perhaps a rougher and readier one is better.

JANE ALLESLEV (Queen's University, Kingston, Ontario): I'd like to ask Dr. Banister this: It appears that you were using the international code to code your diseases and if you were, would you comment on what you will do with the records if the next revision is as drastic as the last one was?

DR. BANISTER: We have the written description of the anomaly and we'll just have to go back and record them as we did this time.

DR. HOOK: I wonder if Dr. Miller might discuss further what flaws in the NINDS study led them to miss the rubella epidemic.

DR. R. MILLER: One reason is that there are only 6,000 patients entered in the study a year -- a relatively small number -- and among those in 1964, only 10 or 12 with rubella syndrome were identified. An additional problem was the

diverse nature of the syndrome which causes
recognition difficulties. But the blood that
NINDS collected was invaluable in relating subtle
effects of rubella infection to the outcome of
the pregnancy. Still another problem was the
time lag. Coding the material takes such a long
time that even if the system did work a cluster
of cases wouldn't be known for some time.

IV. MONITORING MINOR MALFORMATIONS

MINOR MALFORMATIONS:
THEIR RELEVANCE AND SIGNIFICANCE

David W. Smith

Minor anomalies are defined as morphological features which are of no serious medical or cosmetic consequence to the patient. Their recognition can be important since they may serve as indicators of altered morphogenesis in a general sense by alerting the physician to the possibility of a more serious defect in the patient, or in a more specific sense as valuable clues in the diagnosis of a particular known pattern of malformation.

Marden, Smith and McDonald[1] examined a series of 4,412 newborn Caucasian babies for the frequency and nature of minor as well as major malformations. No alteration which was found in more than 4% of the babies was classified as a minor anomaly. Each baby was examined completely, but no attempt was made to determine anomalies of dermal ridge patterning or umbilical cord. Seventy percent of the minor defects noted were of the face, including the ears, and of the hands, areas of relatively complex and variable surface features. The frequency of major defects was 2% with one-third of these babies having multiple major defects. One or more minor anomalies were found in 15% of the babies. Figure 1 contrasts

the frequency of major malformation in relation
to the number of minor anomalies found per baby.
One minor anomaly is of relatively little significance, two are of concern and three or more minor
anomalies in the same baby should create serious
concern about such an infant having a major malformation problem. Judging from this study,
there is value in detecting minor anomalies and
the finding of three or more in the same baby is
usually indicative of a more serious problem in
morphogenesis.

Probably the greatest value of detecting minor
anomalies is in the diagnosis of specific known
syndromes of malformation. Since it is rare for
a given anomaly to be pathognomonic for a given
disorder, the diagnosis of multiple defect
syndromes is generally dependent upon the recognition of a pattern of associated defects. In this
regard, the detection of minor defects enhances
the capacity to arrive at a specific diagnosis.
For example, of the usual anomalies detected at
birth in patients with the autosomal trisomy
syndromes, over half of the defects are minor
ones.

The question is often raised as to which minor
anomalies should especially alert the physician
to do a chromosome study in a patient who has
multiple defects without a clear diagnosis.
Comparing the findings in 11 known chromosomal
abnormality syndromes, as contrasted to the
remaining 124 recognizable patterns of malformation in Smith's[2] textbook, there is no one
anomaly which is found only in chromosomal abnormality syndromes. However, there are several
listed in Table I which may be found in over half
of the chromosomal abnormality syndromes and are
relatively uncommon in known malformation disorders of other modes of etiology.

Besides being important clues in the detection

of major defects and in the diagnosis of specific
syndromes, minor anomalies may be of value in
attempting to determine whether a defect such as
mental deficiency had its onset in prenatal life.
Smith and Bostian[3] found that 42% of a group of
50 children with idiopathic mental deficiency had
three or more associated malformations whereas
none of the 100 control children in that study
had 3 anomalies. The obvious implication is that
the mental deficiency in those children with
several associated anomalies was due to the same
unknown cause as the malformations, and was of
prenatal onset.

A few comments are merited about the nature of
some of the minor anomalies, many of which are
illustrated in the textbook by Smith.[2] First, it
is important to determine whether a given minor
anomaly in the patient is a familial feature or
not. This is especially important for inner
epicanthal fold, clinodactyly of the fifth finger,
simian crease and partial syndactyly between the
second and third toes, each of which may occasionally be familial. Secondly, caution should be
exercised in the diagnosis of a given feature as
a minor malformation. For example, slight inner
epicanthal folds in early infancy should not be
classified as a minor anomaly. Occular hyper-
telorism is rather rare and should be validated
by measurements since a low nasal bridge often
facilitates the visual impression of hyper-
telorism. The ear should only be classified as
low set when the upper helix meets the cranium at
a point below that of a horizontal plane with the
corner of the orbit. Clinodactyly of the fifth
finger is only significant when there is 8 degrees
or more in inturning of the distal fifth finger
as compared to its main axis.

The dermal ridge patterns, dermatoglyphics and
the crease patterns of the hand have been in-

creasingly utilized as indicators of altered
morphogenesis. It is interesting to view both of
these features from a developmental standpoint.
The studies of Mulvihill and Smith[4] indicate that
the parallel dermal ridges of the hand develop
transversely to the lines of growth stress. At
the time of their development, between the 13th
and 19th week of gestation, there are usually
prominent pads on the fingertips and interdigital
areas. The surface topography at that time
affects the patterning of the dermal ridges. Thus,
it is implied that low fetal fingertip pads would
give rise to low arch fingertip patterns such as
found in the 18 Trisomy syndrome and high pads
could give rise to whorl patterns such as are frequently found in XO Turner's syndrome. Furthermore, any gross hand malformation will be
associated with almost predictable secondary
alterations in dermal ridge patterning. The
studies of Popich and Smith[5] indicate that hand
creases reflect the early flexional planes of
folding in the volar skin of the developing hand
between the 9th and 14th week of life. For
example, a lack of development of movement at a
joint will be associated with a lack of crease
development. Thus, the dermal ridge and crease
patterns of the hand are always secondary features providing an indelible historical record of
the early form and surface topography of the hand
in the case of ridge patterns and the form and
flexional function of the early fetal hand in the
case of creases. Abnormalities in dermal ridge
or crease patterns should be interpreted with respect to the more primary anomaly, when possible.

When interpreting any anomaly it is always
important to think in terms of primary defects.
For example, an otherwise normal patient with a
missing thumb, altered dermal ridge patterns in
the thenar area of the palm, and a missing thenar

crease has but one <u>primary</u> anomaly in the development of the thumb and should <u>not</u> be viewed as a multiple defect patient.

A word of caution. There is a tendency to over-interpret minor variations in form as minor anomalies, especially in the newborn baby. The author recommends that you avoid the borderline situations and only accept those features which are quite definitely abnormal as minor anomalies.

REFERENCES

1. Marden, P., Smith, D.W. and McDonald, M.J.: Congenital anomalies in the newborn infant, including minor anomalies. J. Pediat. 64:357, 1964.
2. Smith D.W.: <u>Recognizable Patterns of Human Malformation</u>. W.B.Saunders Company, Philadelphia, 1970.
3. Smith, D.W. and Bostian, K.E.: Congenital anomalies associated with idiopathic mental retardation. J. Pediat. 65:189, 1964.
4. Mulvihill, J.J. and Smith D.W.: The genesis of dermatoglyphics. J. Pediat. 75:579, 1969.
5. Popich, G. and Smith, D.W.: The genesis and significance of digital and palmar flexion creases. J. Pediat. In press, October, 1970.

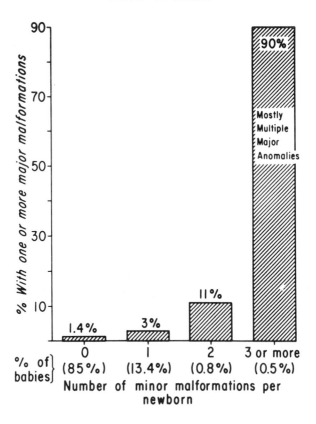

Figure 1. Relative frequency of major malformations in relation to the number of minor anomalies found in each baby. From Marden et al: J.Pediat. 64:357, 1964.

Table 1*

Anomalies which are relatively common in known chromosomal abnormality syndromes versus known patterns of malformation of other etiologies.

SLANTED PALPEBRAL FISSURES

LOOSE FOLDS, POSTERIOR NECK (NEWBORN)

LOW SET EARS

DISTAL PALMAR TRIRADIUS & SIMIAN CREASE

*The anomalies are listed in decreasing order of potential value as possible indicators of a chromosomal abnormality.

SOME GENERAL CONSIDERATIONS CONCERNING MONITORING: APPLICATION TO UTILITY OF MINOR DEFECTS AS MARKERS

Ernest B. Hook

One approach to surveillance is to record phenomena not significant in themselves but which still reflect the effects of environmental insults to the developing fetus. Minor birth defects would appear to be plausible candidates for such markers. These may be defined as human morphological anatomical variations which are of no clinical or cosmetic significance per se, but which occur in higher frequency in individuals with some malformation syndrome than in ostensibly normal infants. This definition is slightly different from that of Marden et al[1] in that it does not exclude a morphological variant as a "defect" simply because it has a high background incidence in normal infants.

There are at least two categories of minor defects that can be studied relatively easily in the newborns. One includes the variation best exemplified by dermatoglyphic patterns -- the ridges on soles, palms and fingers -- and which requires magnification for recording. The other, to which this discussion is restricted, includes malformations grossly visible to the eye.*

---

*The feasibility of dermatoglyphic patterns as markers is discussed on page 199.

On the basis of the relative frequency of some of the apparently more objective malformations we have explored the possibility that screening for selected minor birth defects could be done by relatively unskilled observers who could be trained to search for objective malformations. Furthermore since most minor birth defects of interest occur on the head, face, and hands it appeared that many newborn infants could be quickly examined and scored by such observers since babies would not have to be particularly disturbed in their bassinets.

Over the past year a study of the feasibility of this approach has been carried out in two hospitals in the Albany area. From November 1, 1969 to August 30, 1970 over 3000 consecutive ostensibly normal newborn infants have been examined for the presence of specific defects. These examinations were performed by two laboratory technicians after a two month period of training in newborn evaluation, examination of infants, and scoring of gross minor birth defects. Neither of these individuals had any clinical experience before the start of the investigation. We attempted to score defects which seemed sufficiently objective and frequent ($> 10^{-3}$) to be useful. (Table 1) Of these, five have been retained for definitive scoring and four are still being investigated to establish precise diagnostic criteria. Diagnostic agreement between the two observers for the five defects scored is over 99%.

Once the methodology for scoring and collecting markers had been established, we initiated a structured interview of the mothers of all ostensibly normal infants concerning caffeine ingestion and exposure to one other possible teratogen during gestation. In addition data relating to maternal age, birth weight, race,

178

ethnic status (in some cases), as well as other
population variables has been routinely recorded
from the charts. This was essentially a pilot
study, which was introduced as much to evaluate
our methodology and approach to monitoring as to
evaluate the possible teratogenic effect of any
particular agent. Another purpose was to define
the population variables (in addition to the suspected teratogens) that affect the incidence of
minor defects.

Our working hypothesis has been that selected
minor defects are plausible teratogenic markers.
(The rationale for this assumption is discussed
below.) Assuming a favorable outcome for the
ongoing pilot studies one might visualize a
general monitoring scheme in which, at several
satellite centers, ostensibly normal newborn infants are systematically examined for minor birth
defects while simultaneously their mothers are
queried concerning relevant population factors as
well as exposure to possible teratogens. The
results would then be sent to a central analysis
unit.

How likely is this proposal to meet the re-
quisites of a useful monitoring method? Crow has
proposed six criteria by which approaches to
monitoring for mutations might be evaluated.[2]
These may be slightly modified (Table 2) and
applied to any more general scheme such as the
one proposed here.

1. Relevance. As already indicated, minor
birth defects are not in themselves clinically
significant. Nevertheless, there is reason
to think they are positively correlated with
significant fetal pathology. There are
three lines of evidence for this: a) By
definition an anatomical variant is not classified
as a defect unless it occurs in higher frequency
in some multiple malformation syndrome than in

normal infants, b) As shown by Smith and
Bostian,[3] there is a high incidence of associated
minor defects in an individual with a ventricular
septal defect, even when this is the sole major
malformation. This is of particular interest
since this congenital heart lesion at birth is
frequently cryptic and cannot be diagnosed until
later in infancy. Similarly, idiopathic mental
retardation has a very high incidence of associated minor birth defects.[3] Other evidence that
minor malformations are indicators of subtle
pathology of the central nervous system is
provided by one report that in an otherwise
normal group of two and a half year old children,
the number and severity of minor birth defects
were positively correlated with hyperkinetic,
aggressive, and intractable behavior.[4] c) Rubella,
the best known human teratogen is known to produce an increase in at least one of the minor
defects surveyed, namely, simian lines.[5] Thalidomide, on the basis of one anecdotal report,
also appears to produce simian lines.[6] Epicanthal folds, single flexion creases, simian lines,
and "excrescences" of the ears have been seen in
at least one child with amethopterin embryopathy.[7]

2. Speed of detection. These defects are
all superficial, so may be diagnosed immediately
after birth. They probably reflect fetal
insults in the first three or four months of
gestation. Therefore, the effect of a cryptic
teratogen would be expected to appear from
5 to 9 months after its introduction to the
environment. Thus, this system would be at least
as rapid as a (germinal) mutation monitoring
scheme. In addition, since the marker is
detected before discharge of the infant from the
hospital, rechecking to avoid confusion of cases
may be easily done. In contrast, markers such as
chromosome breaks or biochemical mutations are un-

likely to be detected until after discharge of
the infant.

3. Sensitivity to a small increase in incidence
rate. Crow has suggested that any test system
would have to be applied on a sufficiently large
scale so that any moderate increase in rate, a
doubling or less, could be detected.

One of the main advantages of minor birth
defects compared to other possible markers is
their high incidence, since the more frequent
the marker the smaller the population that has to
be screened to detect significant changes. The
implications of this are illustrated in Table 3.

4. Likelihood of identifying cause of increase.
Suppose there was a significant change in
the incidence of minor defects. This could have
at least three possible explanations. 1) It
could be due to variation in diagnosing cases or
finding cases. In other words the ascertainment
of the system could be changed. 2) There could
be some sudden shift in the population due to
migration or else more subtle shifts in the make-
up of the child bearing population relating to
variables such as parental age, socio-enconomic
status etc., which indirectly may affect the incidence of marker defects. Such effects can be
said to be due to "population" changes. 3) Lastly,
such changes could of course be due to changes in
teratogens or mutagens in the environment. These
may be defined simply as "environmental" causes.

Clearly all three of these are interconnected.
Changes in the population could lead to changes
in ascertainment particularly if not all hospitals
in a community are being surveyed. Changes in
population patterns could also lead to differential exposure of parts of the population to
already existing environmental hazards. Indeed
such population factors as socio-economic status

or parental age, if correlated with differences
in incidence of rate of defects, may already be
indirect reflections of consistent differences in
environmental exposure of particular segments of
population.

One cannot anticipate in advance the a priori
likelihood that any monitoring scheme can identify
the cause of an increased frequency in the marker
employed. Clearly each approach will have
separate specific problems relating to the methodology of marker identification and characterization. However, one can at least compare the
relative chances of any approach since the strategy for identifying population and/or environmental causes once markers are identified are
likely to be the same or quite similar. For
these purposes one can distinguish markers which
are likely to reflect agents acting during gestation and those which indicate earlier effects,
predominantly germinal mutations (in the broad
sense.) We may more simply define these as gestational or pregestational markers.

Chromosome breaks in somatic cells, mosaicism
for protein markers, and chromosomal mosaicism
(particularly XY/XO and XX/XO) are likely to
reflect primarily gestational events. The other
chromosome errors and non-mosaic protein changes
are likely to be indicators of pregestational
events. There are of course exceptions to this
general classification: i.e. the chromosome
breaks in a carrier of Bloom's syndrome may indirectly reflect a recent germinal mutation. But
it seems likely that the magnitude of such mis-
classifications are likely to be small.

It is harder to classify such indicators as
birth defects, prematurity (and/or low birth
weight), fetal wastage, and secondary sex ratio.
For these one must not only try to estimate the
extent to which gestational and pregestational

factors contribute to the "background" rate, but also the likelihood that a <u>rise</u> in incidence can be attributed to one or the other category. It seems likely that, while genetic factors make significant contributions to the background of all four of the markers indicated, changes are likely to reflect primarily gestational events. The grounds for this will be discussed here only as applied to birth defects.

While there are a number of malformation syndromes such as Apert's syndrome, achondroplasia, etc. which appear to be inherited as typical mendelian traits, these are individually quite rare. The chromosomal syndromes associated with malformation are more frequent, but even here the total contribution is not large, and more importantly, the distinctive phenotypes usually enable identification of the error involved. However, the vast bulk of malformations both in quantity and type appear likely to be multifactorial in origin. This appears true not only for major defects but for many minor malformations as well.[8]

Under this hypothesis, manifestation of an anomaly results from the presence of 1) polygenes each of relatively small effect and all of which increase predisposition to defect, and 2) usually unknown environmental factors. There are a number of models but for these purposes, we will consider only that of Carter.[9] This postulates that as a prerequisite for manifestation an individual must have a sufficient number of polygenes affecting predisposition to push him beyond a hypothesized threshold. If over the threshold, the presence of (deleterious) environmental influences will determine whether and to what extent he is affected.

Assuming this model holds for most birth defects, it seems likely that (germinal) mutations are relatively unlikely to play a significant role in any observed large increase in frequency of defects since each gene is of relatively small effect. That is, mutation in polygenes would produce only "quantum" jumps in predisposition (and not necessarily in the required direction). On the other hand, gestational environmental factors could have a marked effect either by lowering the threshold markedly or inducing the defect in those already over the threshold who would not otherwise have been affected. In other words, multifactorial traits seem likely to be more sensitive to abrupt changes in relevant gestational environmental factors than to pregestational mutations in polygenes and, thus, are probably primarily markers of gestational events.

This is an admittedly intuitive argument and not without objection. For instance, an increase of any magnitude in a relevant polygene will still throw a certain fraction of the population over the threshold with concomitant increase in rate affected. Secondly, while the direction of any mutation cannot be predicted a priori, it seems likely that a random mutation will result in loss or diminished function of the gene involved with resultant diminished developmental stability, i.e., in direction towards the threshold for the defect. Thirdly, the threshold itself may be lowered by a mutation in a major gene. Nevertheless, considering 1) the well-documented effects of a teratogen such as rubella in producing sudden increases in major defects usually regarded as multifactorial in humans, and 2) the lack of evidence that new mutations have ever been responsible for an abrupt rise in the rate or a difference in rate between populations for any significant fraction of such traits, the original argument appears plausible.

It seems likely that, other things being equal,

a gestational indicator will be more useful for determining the cause of any increase in incidence. At the time of ascertainment one is temporally closer to the presumed cause. Exposure to possibly relevant environmental factors is likely to be far better recalled by the parents. Other information concerning drugs, X-rays, etc., are available from medical records describing the course of the pregnancy. And of course (in the first analysis at least) the environmental exposure of only the mother need be scrutinized, vastly simplifying the range of factors to be considered and eliminating concern with possible illegitimacy. In contrast, for pregestational markers there will be at least a nine month and possibly a much longer lag (with the exception of markers in abortuses or amniotic fluid) between the time of environmental insult and detection of the effect. In addition interviews of both parents will have to be done. (The only exception to this might be for a marker such as the XYY karyotype which is attributable to a paternal germinal event. Such indicators are quite rare.)

The other distinction that might be made is between a catastrophic phenotypic marker and a subtle one. This relates to the reliability of information extracted from parental interview. It is well known that a mother of an infant with a marked congenital malformation is likely to have an acute, even a "hyperacute" memory for all possibly relevant factors during or before gestation compared to a mother of an ostensibly normal baby. In addition interviews done systematically shortly after the event are likely to be delicate and possibly traumatic. But use of a marker without marked phenotypic effect avoids these difficulties.

Thus the gestational indicators with subtle

effect appear to be the most promising for
identifying likely causes of increased marker
frequency. Somatic mutations, chromosome breaks
and minor defects fall in this category.

5. Sensitivity to multiple causes. As already
discussed, minor birth defects may be produced by
rubella, thalidomide and amethopterin, quite dis-
tinct teratogens whose spectrum of effect does
not usually overlap to a large extent. This, in
conjunction with the already noted extensive
association of these minor birth defects with a
wide variety of other malformation syndromes as
extensively documented in Smith's monograph,[10]
suggests that they are relatively non-specific
indicators of fetal insult.

There are a few generalizations one can make in
comparing the sensitivity of pregestational and
gestational markers to environmental insult. An
agent that induces germinal mutations is
highly likely to produce somatic mutations in
embryonic cells as well. This or other factors
may explain why almost all mutagens appear to be
teratogens also. But the converse is not true.
Thus monitoring for gestational events will be
sensitive to a much wider variety of environmental insults than monitoring just for pregestational events.

6. Availability. In the sense in which Crow
defines this term, minor birth defects are close
to being "available" for a monitoring system. The
one remaining question concerns comparability of
data from separate centers. It is likely that
any single unit is likely to be consistent in its
diagnostic evaluation. This would probably
apply even to relatively subjective defects such
as low placed ears, for which it is notoriously
difficult to devise precise and easily diagnostic
criteria in the newborn. But even with what we
have classified as the objective minor birth

defects, there are occasional borderline situations (albeit less than 1%) which are difficult to classify. We have drawn up what we regard as precise diagnostic criteria for the defects employed and believe we have been consistent in their use. But demonstrating their adequacy requires compilation of a complete atlas of all variations of such defects for evaluation of criteria. This is in progress, although it is difficult to anticipate with such a collection every possible anatomical variant that can arise.

One way of avoiding at least part of this difficulty would be to establish a diagnostic center to which satellite centers could send photographs of all infants in whom a defect was even suspected. This would allow a greater tolerance in diagnostic skill in the peripheral examiners as well as eliminate any difficulty in comparing results within or between centers. Such an approach would also allow a single systematic approach to scoring some of the relatively more subjective defects such as malformed or asymmetric ears. Of course use of photographic recording would raise the cost of this approach. A cheaper method would be simply to train all examiners at the same location before they went out to satellite centers, and periodically re-examine them with test atlases to be sure diagnostic standards were not changing.

7. _Cost_. The cost of monitoring minor birth defects can be estimated making the following assumptions: 1) A minimum of 50,000 individuals nationally should be evaluated per year; 2) ten satellite centers could evaluate 50,000 to 100,000 infants per year; 3) each center could be manned by two full time individuals with an additional part time person; 4) the average salary per technician would be

about $9,000 per year, and 5) the additional costs of data collection would run a maximum of $1,000 per year per hospital. The total estimated cost of data collection would then be about $250,000. Possibly this might be cut close to half by only interviewing mothers when a rise in incidence was observed. In any event, in view of the order of magnitude of funds involved, it would appear wise not to attempt to initiate this approach on a large scale until at least pilot studies had actually revealed a teratogen using this approach.

Of course, it is likely that once that any particular monitoring system is set up, others can be integrated fairly easily. For instance, monitoring 50,000 to 100,000 infants per year for minor birth defects by direct inspection will lend itself relatively easily to monitoring for major defects by direct inspection as well. Thus, one would not have to depend on medical records or birth certificates which are notoriously difficult to use for such purposes. Other variables which could easily be evaluated are prematurity and head circumference. In addition, cord bloods could be frozen and a selected portion analyzed for biochemical mutations should there be an abrupt increase in rate of gestational markers analyzed.

ACKNOWLEDGEMENTS

I thank Dong-Soo Kim, Judith Jackson Petry, M. Linda Powers and Lynda Hess for assistance and stimulation in these studies; I.H. Porter for encouragement; and the medical and nursing staffs at Albany Medical Center and St. Peter's Hospital for their cooperation.

REFERENCES

1. Marden, P.M., Smith, D.W. and McDonald, M.J.: Congenital anomalies in the newborn infant, including minor variations. J. Pediat. 64: 357, 1964.

2. Crow, J.F.: Human population monitoring, chapter in Environmental Chemical Mutagens. A. Hollaender, ed., Plenum Press, (in press).

3. Smith, D.W. and Bostian, K.E.: Congenital anomalies associated with idiopathic mental retardation. J. Pediat. 65: 189, 1964.

4. Waldrop, M.F., Pederson, F.A. and Bell, R.Q.: Minor physical anomalies and behavior in pre-school children. Child. Dev. 39: 391, 1968.

5. Achs, R., Harper, R.G. and Siegel, M.: Unusual dermatoglyphic findings associated with rubella embryopathy. New Eng. J. Med. 274: 148, 1966.

6. Davies, P. and Smallpiece, V.: The single transverse palm crease in infants and children. Develop. Med. Child. Neurol. 5: 491, 1963.

7. Milunsky, A., Graet, J.W. and Gaynor, M.F.: Methotrexate induced congenital malformations. J. Pediat. 72: 790, 1968.

8. Hook, E. B., Powers, M.L. and Kim, D.S.: In preparation.

9. Carter, C.O.: Multifactorial inheritance revisited, in Congenital Malformations, Proc. 3rd Int. Conf., Excerpta Medica, Amsterdam, 1970,

p. 227.
10. Smith, D.W.: Recognizable Patterns of Human Malformations. W. B. Saunders, Philadelphia, 1970,
11. National Institutes of Environmental Health Sciences: Report of the committee for the study of monitoring of human mutagenesis. (H.E.Sutton, Chairman). See p. 275.

Table 1

Approximate incidence of selected minor defects
(x 10^{-3}) in Albany newborn without major defects

lack of helical fold	35
markedly asymmetric ears +	1
severely slanting ears +	2
ear pits +	2
Sydney lines	50
clinodactyly +	10
epicanthal folds *	25
simian creases *	20
bridged creases *	50
single flexion crease *	1
ear tags *	3

*currently monitored
+under investigation (see text)

Table 2

Crow's Criteria for Monitoring Systems (Modified)

1. Relevance
2. Speed of detection
3. Sensitivity to small increase in incidence
4. Sensitivity to multiple causes
5. Likelihood of identifying cause of increase
6. Availability
7. Cost

Table 3

Sensitivity of Various Markers to Change in Incidence ‡

Defect	"Objective" minor birth defects	Most frequent minor (simian lines)	All major (recognizable at birth)	Most frequent major (club feet)	Most frequent useful major (cleft lip)	All detectable mutations (10 systems)	Single mutations
Frequency per newborn	.10	.07-.05	~.02	~.006	~.002	.0002	.00002
Doubling denominator *	455	673-979	2581	8811	26,611	267,000	2,670,000
Smallest % detectable increase +							
10^6 births	.6%	.7%-.9%	1.4%	2.6%	4.4%	14%	40%
10^5 births	1.9%	2.3%-2.8%	4.4%	8.1%	12.1%	44.7%	141.4%

* The population required to reveal a doubling in incidence ($\beta=.95$), p <.01, assuming homogeneous composition.

+ The smallest percent increase in a scored marker producing a rise beyond the 95% confidence interval of baseline frequency, calculated using the normal approximation to the binomial distribution.

‡ These comparisons of the "power" of marker incidence do not necessarily reflect differences in marker sensitivity to environmental effects.

DISCUSSION

DR. KARL S. WITTMAN (Hudson Valley Community College, Troy, New York): I wonder if Dr. Smith would comment on how parentally transmitted genetic background might affect the incidence of defects in terms of expressivity or penetrance of the gene.

DR. SMITH: In relation to family histories, if we find a person with an anomaly which is also present in other members of his family, (and sometimes this can be seen over several generations) that anomaly is assumed to be a normal variant in that particular family. But, in general, we cannot distinguish a single gene effect from a multiple one.

DR. HOOK: We have tried to investigate the extent of this type of "noise" with regard to simian lines and epicanthal folds in our population here. In about 2,000 mother-infant pairs, we have not found a significant increase in the frequency of affected babies born to mothers with a malformation as compared to babies born to unaffected mothers. Of course, the number of mothers affected is fairly small. I am sure that there is a strong genetic component to these defects. We are unable to detect it at present.

DR. FRASER: I'd like to comment on Dr. Hook's comments about minor malformations (anomalies) in children known to have been exposed to teratogenic agents. In most of the examples cited, as in the case of thalidomide and amethopterin, major malformations occur as well. It's not too surprising that thalidomide children have dermatoglyphic anomalies in hands that may have digital anomalies. I wonder if anyone is looking at children who have been exposed in utero to other

kinds of teratogenic agents. For instance: PKU
mothers whose children don't have major malformations but might have the minor ones -- there
are an appreciable number of such children around
though I don't know of any data on them; secondly,
perhaps, those exposed to progestational agents,
although this might be too limited to the genito-
urinary system; thirdly, those exposed to intrauterine radiation. In mice at least, something
as low as 5 R will produce demonstrable minor
anomalies. It might be worthwhile looking at
children from this point of view.

DR. HOOK: I agree completely. Clearly, phocomelia is a much better sign of thalidomide embryopathy than simian lines. On the other hand, it's
possible that for other teratogens, such as
rubella, the minor birth defects might, in fact,
be relatively good as subtle markers.

DR. LAWRENCE R. SHAPIRO (Letchworth Village,
Thiells, New York): Dr. Smith, if one considers
the dermatoglyphic patterns to be related to
morphogenesis, or variability of morphogenesis
during gestation, how does one account for the
persistent patterns of decreased total ridge
count in certain chromosomal anomalies as in
trisomy 18?

DR. SMITH: In the trisomy 18 syndrome, there
is hypoplasia of many individual organ structures.
I consider the low arch digital pattern to be an
indicator of hypoplasia of the fetal fingertip
pads.
  I would like to bring out one point about the
minor anomalies in general -- they are relatively
non-specific indicators of altered morphogenesis,
but, in some respects, they may be valuable. I
don't think you'll get any specificity out of

observing a single crease on the upper palm or in-
turned fifth finger, but they may be non-specific
indicators of altered morphogenesis so your
scrutiny is far better if you include minor anomalies rather than if you deal just with major
defects. However, I think it needs to be appre-
ciated that it's going to be a non-specific kind
of scrutiny.

DR. SKALKO: I'd like to make a reference to
the use of syndromes to determine which environmental agent is operative in producing congenital
malformations. If you define a syndrome with
respect to a particular teratogen, as for example,
either trypan blue or hypervitaminosis A in rats,*
where the syndromes are different and then com-
bine these two non-related teratogens, you get a
syndrome that is completely different and it is
not possible to determine which of the two, or
their interactions produced the specific malformation that you see. So, when working with a
multifactorial system, as Dr. Hook has pointed
out, it is extremely difficult to get at a
specific environmental cause. From experimental
evidence we know we can produce a completely
different syndrome with two specific environmental
insults, therefore, in the human population, we
have no way of knowing how many insults are, in
fact, related to a specific malformation.

DR. SUTTON: It seems to me that there exists
the same problems here that have been discussed
in relation to mutagenesis, in trying to monitor
by sentinel phenotypes. In order to have a useful monitoring system, you somehow need to
determine which phenotypes represent noise. In
other words, in a genetic system you have to

---

*Wilson, J.G., Anat. Rec. 142:292, 1962.

account for those that were inherited from the parents in order to identify those which are, in fact, new mutations. A system may well show mutation but unless one out of every hundred, or one out of every thousand such cases is, in fact, a mutant, then it is not a useful system with which to monitor mutagenesis. I would raise the same question with respect to those minor malformations which have a high frequency. Let us suppose, for example, that these minor malformations occur in 10% of the population and that at least 90% of that is genetic. I think your calculations are based on the assumption that all of the 10% is due to a single cause and that the number you'd need to detect an increase are all also due to the same cause. Since I am not a teratologist, perhaps someone else, more involved in this area, would like to comment on it, as I am uncomfortable about it.

DR. HOOK: Lack of knowledge of the exact magnitude of the genetic component of a teratogenic marker does complicate interpretation of the doubling denominator, since, even assuming linear and equal responses to the environmental teratogenic causes, more than a doubling in the background dose of these offending agents may be required to produce a doubling in incidence of the defect. On the other hand, an observed abrupt rise in incidence in a multifactorial trait is highly likely to have a <u>single</u> specific environmental cause. But, in a practical sense, perhaps the only real answer to your question will come from pilot studies to see if we can identify a teratogenic effect of a compound, producing a rise, perhaps, of only 10% to 11%, using minor defects as a marker.

Would that satisfy your objections or do you think there would be further problems?

DR. SUTTON: I think, in terms of practice, it doesn't quite satisfy the problem. The small increase may, indeed, reflect the effect of an environmental agent, but it is difficult to determine which part of the small increase is due to an environmental agent and which is due to variance in the background, which has a relatively high base frequency.

DR. HOOK: But that is a problem with any marker, even point mutations. As long as the background rate is greater than zero, given an abrupt rise in incidence it will be difficult to distinguish which particular observed cases are due to the background and which to a postulated new environmental insult. All would have to be investigated to pick up the factor that may be responsible for only a proportion of new cases. By continually monitoring a population, however, if the abrupt rise occurs at the same time that there is a change in a relevant environmental variable, one will have at least a working hypothesis on which to focus in investigating the entire group.

THE POSSIBLE VALUE OF DERMATOGLYPHIC RIDGE PATTERNS AND ASYMMETRY AS TERATOGENIC MARKERS

Ernest B. Hook

Dermatoglyphic ridge patterns have been widely studied in major malformation syndromes.[1] However, with one possible exception (see below) their utility as general markers of environmental insult has not been previously considered. Of course there are a number of specific limitations upon their use. While there are over 20 separate regions on the hand and foot where one can look for patterns and a great variety of patterns that can occur in these regions, it is not at all clear which particular findings can be regarded as signs of a generalized fetal insult. In the sense already defined (see p. 177) only a few variants can be regarded as a minor birth "defect" and these tend to be relatively specific for an associated major malformation syndrome. Thus multiple arches are a sign of Trisomy 18 syndrome (or 3 additional X chromosomes) but there is no evidence that an individual with multiple arches but without a rare chromosomal error is much more likely to have phenotypic damage, cryptic or otherwise, than an individual chosen randomly.

There is only one exception to this: the location of the distal most axial triradius on the palms. The placement of this triradius (labeled t, t' or t" depending how high it is) can be measured 1) by calculating the angle subtended by it and two other triradii on the palm, the a and d, (angle), 2) by measuring the ratio of the distance of the t triradius from the most distal wrist crease to the distance from this crease to the most proximal crease at the base of the 3rd or 4th finger, (ratio) or 3) by counting the number of ridges between it and the d triradius (ridge). With any method, the greater the measurement, the higher the triradius and the more likely this sign is to reflect fetal maldevelopment.

An elevated triradius is not only the most ubiquitous dermatoglyphic finding in the chromosomal syndromes, but is found in other multiple malformation syndromes, idiopathic mental retardation, isolated ventricular septal defect, and cleft lip.[2] And in addition it is one sign of rubella embryopathy[3,4] so that is sensitive to at least one environmental teratogen. Another advantage of using this marker is that its position is a continuous variable. Analysis of a possible correlation with other factors thus is subject to much greater precision.

The main drawback in using this for monitoring is the difficulty in precisely determining its position in the newborn. Since location of the a and d triradius is often difficult and ridge counting is practically impossible, the most practical method is calculating the ratio. But flexion creases are not the best landmarks and a certain error in observation is introduced. And for large scale monitoring one must have a method that is not only reliable but also quick. Unfortunately, the hand of the newborn is one of the most difficult sources from which to score patterns efficiently and most traditional methods of recording patterns are not successful with the newborn palms.

D.S. Kim and I have tried monitoring axial

triradii in the newborn using simply an illuminated magnifier and recording the triradial
position as "elevated" or "normal." Unfortunately our experience indicates that without
some method for actually recording location,
these remain only subjective judgements.

In our own experience the most useful approach
has been of an inkless dermatoglyphic device
based upon the principle of internal reflection
or else a CU-5 close up camera. These have draw-
backs in that they are, at present state of
development, tedious and cumbersome to use and
somewhat costly. Nevertheless it seems likely
that refinement of these approaches is only a
technical problem and it will only be a matter of
time before more feasible methods are available.
The apparatus will be costly compared to present
techniques but probably no more so than some of
the instrumentations currently used for detection
of mutation or chromosome breaks.

The problem is exactly the opposite with
patterns on the foot of the newborn. It is relatively easy to determine the presence and type
of pattern on the big toe, hallucal area of the
sole, and calcar area, but no ubiquitous sign of
maldevelopment has been noted in these areas.

Even the traditional methods of printing are
often successful here. And since, in New York
State at least, by law the pattern on the foot at
birth must be taken and kept in the chart to
avoid confusion of babies there is a large
reservoir of potential information on file. Unfortunately the law doesn't specify that the
patterns should be legible! Kim and I recently
compared the patterns deciphered from the charts
of newborns with those we noted using illuminated
magnification. The results indicated that for at
least the hallucal and calcar areas, in a surprisingly large number of cases (about 60%) the

charts provided adequate information. The patterns originally had been taken by a large number of individuals. Had all used a reasonable amount of care accuracy would have been much improved. Perhaps changing the law or hospital standards for accreditation would improve the situation.

Nevertheless, the newborn patterns on file in hospitals throughout the country probably constitute one of the largest dermatoglyphic resources available. Should a particular sign on the foot eventually prove to be a non-specific marker of development there will be a large backlog of data with which to study recent temporal trends.

An alternative approach to using specific patterns is to use asymmetry of patterns as markers. It seems plausible that teratogens might vary in effects on left or right sides because of slight differences in fetal blood flow or other local factors affecting lateral manifestation. While this might affect the entire body it is easiest to study asymmetry dermatoglyphically since a number of various patterns can be compared and results analyzed quantitatively. A similar suggestion has been made by others concerning the possibility of asymmetry as a marker for somatic mutations.[5] Some suggestive evidence for their utility here are derived from a case of chromosomal mosaicism in which dermatoglyphic findings of interest (as well as most of the somatic abnormalities) were confined to the left side.[6] But this case appears atypical judging from most other reported chromosomal mosaics(see e.g. ref. 7).

Recently, in collaboration with R. Harper and R. Achs, dermatoglyphic asymmetry was evaluated in rubella embryopathy, using the data from the 20 affected and 20 control infants that had been

the subject of the first investigation of dermatoglyphic patterns in this syndrome.[3] For all
variables investigated: finger patterns, palm
patterns, sole patterns and variance between
sides in triradius location and pattern intensity,
there is no increase in asymmetry.[8] In fact, the
trend for each is in the opposite direction,
suggesting that, contrary to hypothesis, if anything rubella diminishes asymmetry. Perhaps this
is because rubella is a strong teratogen whose
effects override slight pre-existing differences
between sides. Conceivably, a weaker teratogen
might have an opposite effect. Nevertheless, the
observed trends suggest that dermatoglyphic
asymmetry per se does not seem likely to be an
ubiquitous teratogenic marker.

REFERENCES

1. Alter, M. Dermatoglyphics in Birth Defects.
   Birth Defects: Original Series, 5:103, 1969.
2. Smith, D. W. and Bostian, K.E.: Congenital
   anomalies associated with idiopathic mental
   retardation. J. Pediat. 65: 189, 1964.
3. Achs, R., Harper, R. G. and Siegel, M.:
   Unusual dermatoglyphic findings associated
   with rubella embryopathy. New Eng. J. Med.
   274:148, 1966.
4. Alter, M. and Schulenberg, R.: Dermatoglyphics in the rubella syndrome. J. Amer.
   Med. Assn. 197:685, 1966.
5. National Institute of Environmental Health
   Sciences: Report of the committee for the
   study of monitoring human mutagenesis, H.E.
   Sutton, Chairman. (See p. 277 .)
6. Hook, E.B. and Yunis, J.J.: Congenital
   asymmetry associated with trisomy 18 mosaicism. Amer. J. Dis. Child. 110: 551, 1965.
7. Penrose, L.S. and Smith, G.F.: Down's Anom-

aly. J.A. Churchill, Ltd., London, 1966.
p. 74. (Polani and Polani (Ann. Hum. Genet.
32:391, 1969) suggest, in analyzing these
data as well as some of their own, that there
may be at least a statistical increase in
left-right asymmetry in trisomy 21 mosaics
for both maximal atd angle (uncorrected for
age) and total finger ridge count.)
8. Hook, E.B., Harper, R.G. and Achs, R.: An
investigation of dermatoglyphic asymmetry in
rubella embryopathy. Teratology, in press.

V. MONITORING MUTATIONS

SOME PROBLEMS IN THE BIOCHEMICAL APPROACH TO DETECTING HUMAN MUTATIONS*

I. Herbert Scheinberg

Introduction

In his article on "Human Population Monitoring,"
Dr. Crow writes of biochemical monitoring that
the ". . . idea here is to use laboratory methods
to detect altered proteins."[1] The Committee for
the Study of Monitoring Human Mutagenesis recommends support for a screening program for mutations based on such methods.[1] In a 1968 WHO
report[2] recommending monitoring of selected populations for genetic abnormalities, the appropriate biochemical techniques are considered to
include quantitative measurements of proteins and
of metabolic intermediates, in addition to the
detection of qualitatively altered proteins.

Types of Measurements and Materials

Techniques for detecting mutations through
alterations in the structure of the DNA of single

---

*Supported in part by grants from the
National Institute of Arthritis and Metabolic
Disease (AI 01059), National Institute of Neuro-
logic Diseases and Blindness and the National
Genetics Foundation, Inc.

genes do not exist nor are they likely to be developed soon. Metabolic intermediates, generally non-protein, include lipids, carbohydrates, amino acids and such complex derivatives as mucopolysaccharides. Excessive accumulations of normal substances of this type, or of metals, or the appearance of abnormal metabolites can indicate the presence of a pathological mutation as in PKU or Wilson's Disease. Indeed, biochemical measurements of this type are today the most commonly used methods of biochemical screening for hereditary diseases, in part because they are often susceptible to automated analysis. Most have, however, the disadvantage of dependence on a measurement at least one step removed from the primary disorder. Thus, in a clinically normal heterozygous infant, diet may elevate the concentration of phenylalanine into the range found in PKU. In patients with biliary cirrhosis, hepatic copper concentrations may reach the levels seen in Wilson's disease. Consequently, at present, ideal biochemical monitoring for mutations should be restricted to measurements on proteins. Practically, analyses can be made only on cord blood, systemic blood or placentae.

All qualitative differences between allelic proteins, even if only detectable as secondary, tertiary or quaternary structural characteristics, presumably reflect substitution, addition or deletion of specific amino acids in polypeptide chains. Such qualitative differences are most directly -- though not most easily -- demonstrated by sequential analysis of the entire protein or its fragments.

If there is a difference between proteins in their contents of aspartic acid, glutamic acid, histidine, lysine or arginine, free or zone electrophoresis[3,4] is probably the simplest method of distinguishing them. The only electri-

cal measurements which can discriminate between
proteins which differ only in their content of
one or more of the remaining amino acids are those
directed toward the proteins' dipole moments--
i.e. dielectric measurements or dielectrophoresis.

Immunochemical distinctions which may also reflect the differences in amino acid sequences can
be demonstrated by the Ouchterlony technique[5] or
by immunoelectrophoresis.[6]

Finally, chromatographic methods may distinguish genetic variants of the same protein.[7]

For large-scale monitoring of mutations, the
disadvantage of all four of these methods is the
difficulty, or impossibility, of automating them.

Quantitative abnormalities of specific proteins
--which are always deficiencies -- may be determined either by specific chemical -- often enzymatic -- properties of the protein, or by immunochemical analysis.[8] Both types of methods can be
rather readily automated. Unfortunately, however,
though deficiency of a specific protein may be inherited and can be the cause of a specific illness -- as is true of a number of erythrocytic
enzymes (Table I) and plasma proteins (Table II)--
acquired deficiency may make the diagnostic value
of the determination misleading. For example,
life-long deficiency of ceruloplasmin is found in
about 97% of patients with Wilson's disease but a
deficiency of this protein may be observed in
subjects without Wilson's disease who suffer from
massive renal or gastro-intestinal protein loss,
or whose diets are grossly lacking in copper.
Furthermore, because many plasma proteins are
normally deficient or virtually absent at birth
(Table III), cord blood, which is so readily
available in relatively large amounts, is only
suitable for monitoring deficiencies of some
proteins of plasma (Table IV). Very little data
are available on the relative concentrations of

cellular enzymes in cord and adult blood.

The advantages and disadvantages of attempting to monitor human mutations by analyses of blood are summarized in Table V.

A Pilot Program and its Results

From November 1965 through April 1969 a pilot program, devised to determine the feasibility of routinely screening large numbers of children for several genetic disorders, was carried out at the Albert Einstein College of Medicine. "Genetic Alert", as it was called, was supported first, by the National Foundation for Neuromuscular Diseases (now the National Genetics Foundation) and then by the National Institute of Neurological Diseases and Blindness (now the National Institute of Neurological Diseases and Stroke). About 1 ml. of capillary blood was drawn from children, generally between the ages of 6 months and 6 years. Relevant genetic information taken from the mother at the same time, was entered onto punched cards. Automated, quantitative analyses were carried out, chemically, for ceruloplasmin,[2] α-1-antitrypsin and G-6-PD, and immunochemically, for transferrin,[8] immunoglobulins A, G and M, and C_1 esterase inhibitor. The analog outputs of the Autoanalyzers (R) used for the determinations were digitized and automatically entered on punched cards, together with the results of analyses of standards and accuracy controls interspersed among the unknowns. The results were computed and printed out automatically, together with the genetic data, stored, for later retrieval, in the central laboratory and reported to the individual child's clinic (Fig.1).

Some of the quantitative results are summarized in Table VI. The cost of the 3 1/2 year program, including purchase of analytical instruments and rental of computing equipment, was about $350,000.

Approximately 25,000 tests were performed on about 7,000 children.

Summary and Conclusions

Biochemical methods are currently available, or can be readily devised, for monitoring mutations of over a dozen proteins of blood associated with inherited human disease. In some cases, qualitative abnormalities can be detected, and these are generally specific; in other instances, deficiencies of individual proteins can be measured and, though these are less specific because they can be acquired, they are generally susceptible to automated analysis.

A computerized pilot program, in which about 25,000 automated tests for eight proteins were carried out in about 7,000 children, over a 3 1/2 year period, cost about $350,000.

Programs of this sort are capable of expansion in the near future to perhaps several dozen proteins and disorders, and have direct applicability to detecting human mutations and hereditary defects. The computerized data permit distinguishing children with specific hereditary disorders and, stored retrievably, are the basis for estimating the prevalence in the screened population of the specific genetic abnormality for comparison with other populations.

REFERENCES

1. Crow, J.F.: Human population monitoring in Environmental Chemical Mutagens. Edited by A. Hollaender. New York, Plenum Press, (in press) 1970.
2. Screening for inborn errors of metabolism. Wld. Hlth. Org. techn. Rep. Ser., No. 401, 1968.
3. Jaffe, E.R.: Hereditary hemolytic disorders and enzymatic deficiencies of human erythrocytes.

Blood 35: 116-134, 1970.
4. Cited in Schultze, H.E., Heremans, J.F.:
Molecular Biology of Human Proteins. Volume I.
Amsterdam, Elsevier Publishing Company, p.384,
1966.
5. Ibid. p. 402.
6. Ibid. p. 423.
7. Broman, L.: Separation and characterization
of two coeruloplasmins from human serum. Nature
182: 1655-1657, 1958.
8. Eckman, I., Robbins, J.B., Van den Hamer,
C.J.A., et al.: Automation of a quantitative
immunochemical microanalysis of human serum
transferrin: a model system. Clin. Chem. 16:
558-561, 1970.

BIRTH DEFECTS MONITORING

GENETIC ALERT CENTRAL LABORATORY
ALBERT EINSTEIN COLLEGE OF MEDICINE
NEW YORK,N.Y.,10461

RESULTS OF GENETIC ALERT TESTS

PREPARED 12/09/68 FOR
E.174 STREET HEALTH CENTER
BRONX,NEW YORK

NAME -   HOSPITAL CHART NO-
AND -   GENETIC ALERT NO- 580199-1
ADDR.- BX N Y 10460   LABORATORY NO   -   006302

        RACE- NEGRO
        SEX- F   BIRTHDATE- 11/65
        SINGLE BIRTH
        BLOOD SOURCE- CAPILLARY
        DATE BLOOD TAKEN- 10/31/68
        INFORMANT-PARENT

SELECTION BASIS-TESTED AS OUT-PATIENT
                6MOS.&

TEST FOR	SERUM CONCENTRATION	USUAL CONCENTRATION	COMMENTS
CERULOPLASMIN	58 (MG/100 ML)	OVER 20 BELOW 100	
ALPHA-1-TRYPSIN INHIBITOR	0.91 (MG TRYPSIN INHIBITED/ML)	OVER 0.8	
IGG	1442 (MG/100 ML)	OVER 400 BELOW 1500	
TRANSFERRIN	327 (MG/100 ML)	NOT YET DETERMINED	
IGA	95 (MG/100 ML)	DEPENDS ON AGE	
IGM	55 (MG/100 ML)	DEPENDS ON AGE	

Figure 1. Results of Genetic Alert tests in one individual.

I. HERBERT SCHEINBERG

TABLE I

Hereditary Anemias Associated with Abnormalities
or Deficiency of an Erythrocytic Enzyme

Enzyme	Qualitative Abnormality* in	Inheritance
Hexokinase	some patients	AR
Phosphohexose isomerase	all patients	AR
Triosephosphate isomerase	all patients	AR
Phosphoglycerate kinase	?	X
Pyruvate kinase	?	AR
Glutathione synthetase	?	AR
G-6-PD	some patients	X

*Electrophoretic (E.R.Jaffé, Blood, $\underline{35}$:116, 1970)

TABLE II

Some Plasma Proteins Associated with
Inherited Disease

Immune globulins	Pseudocholinesterase
C$_1$-esterase inhibitor	α-1-antitrypsin
Albumin	Ceruloplasmin
Transferrin	Lipoproteins
Clotting components	

(Modified from I.H. Scheinberg in Barnett's Pediatrics, 14th Ed., 1968)

214

BIRTH DEFECTS MONITORING

TABLE III

Some Proteins Present in Human Cord Blood
at Less than Adult Concentrations

α-1-lipoprotein	β_1c-globulin
Haptoglobin	C-reactive protein
Ceruloplasmin	Immunoglobulin A
Low-density lipoprotein	Immunoglobulin M

(Modified from H.E. Schultze and J.F. Heremans, 1966.)

TABLE IV

Some Proteins Present in Human Cord Blood
at Roughly Adult Concentrations

Prealbumin	Hemopexin
Albumin	Transferrin
α-1-antitrypsin	Fibrinogen
Orosomucoid	Immunoglobulin G (of
Thyroxine-binding globulin	maternal origin)
Gc-globulin	α-2-macroglobulin

(Modified from H.E.Schultze and J.F.Heremans,1966)

TABLE V

Detecting a Mutation by Demonstrating a Protein's --

QUALITATIVE ABNORMALITY		DEFICIENCY	
Advantages	Disadvantages	Advantages	Disadvantages
Specific	Methods not easily automated	Methods easily automated	Non-specific
Applicable to cord blood			Often inapplicable to cord blood
Detect heterozygotes			

215

TABLE VI

Analyses for Certain Protein Deficiencies in Genetic Alert Program

Protein	Mode of Inheritance	Number Tested	Period of Testing	Mean	2 S.D.	Number of Positives	Number of False Positives*
Ceruloplasmin	AR	7109	11/65-11/68	51 mg%	36 mg%	76**	67, of which 36 are newborns
α-1-trypsin inhibitor	AR	6821	11/65-11/68	1.14 mg trypsin inhibited per ml.	.42 mg	104***	21
Transferrin	AR	4257	6/67-11/68	272 mg%	162 mg%	Normal value not defined	
IgA	Uncertain	784	8/68-11/68	143 mg%	146 mg%	Normal value not defined	
IgG	Sex-linked	4856	1/67-11/68	969 mg%	696 mg%	50****	18
IgM	Uncertain	498	10/68-11/68	63 mg%	98mg%	Normal value not defined	

* These false positives resulted from insufficient serum, laboratory error on first analysis, or analysis of material which was not undiluted human serum.

** Known Wilson's disease patients; patients with nephrotic syndrome or cystinuria.

*** All presumed heterozygotes.

**** 26 males with hereditary or acquired deficiency; 24 females with presumed acquired deficiency.

PROSPECTS FOR THE AUTOMATED TYPING OF BIOCHEMICAL MARKERS FOR THE PURPOSE OF MONITORING THE HUMAN GERMINAL MUTATION RATE

Lowell Weitkamp

The existence of a protein implies the existence of at least one genetic locus and the occurrence of a genetically determined variant of a protein, the occurrence of at least one variant allele, once upon a time a new mutant. At present there is no more directly relevant way to monitor changes in the germinal mutation rate than by determining changes in the frequency of mutant proteins in the population. Heritable protein variants are detectable by a variety of electrophoretic, quantitative and immunologic techniques, each with a different potential for the detection of new mutants and also for adaptation to mechanized or automated systems.

SELECTION OF A SCREENING TECHNIQUE

Immunologic techniques -- such as those which have been successfully used to recognize the allelic variability in the Gm, Inv, Ag, Lp and Xm protein systems -- are suitable for the purpose of screening for mutant proteins. They are inefficient in that the variability recognized may be confined to 1 or 2% of the protein molecule and impracticable in that the recognition of a variant by direct typing requires an antiserum specific for the particular variant in question.

Quantitative analysis performed in solution is particularly adaptable to rapid mechanized procedures. As an example, the Bausch and Lomb Zymat 340 Enzyme Analyzer is capable of the quantitation of the activity of any enzyme which can be coupled to the oxidation or reduction of NAD or NADP. The machine is automatic from the point of withdrawing a measured amount of sample to the graphical display of the curve of the change in absorbance versus the change in time and is capable of processing one sample every two minutes. Using a similar type of analyzer built from commercially available Auto Analyzer modules, Eckman et al.[1] have determined the quantity of transferrin in 100 μl serum samples by measuring the turbidity following the addition of goat antihuman transferrin. The apparatus can process one sample per minute, and an estimated standard deviation from the true value of 7.9 mg% (normal range is 200-300 mg%) indicates the method is accurate. Importantly, the technique is potentially adaptable to any protein; the authors report that it has already been utilized to measure five serum proteins simultaneously, from C 1 esterase inhibitor with a concentration of 25 mg% to IgG with a concentration of 2000 mg%. A new "fast" analyzer has been developed by Anderson[2] using centrifugal force to measure and transfer liquids in a multiple cuvette rotor. The rotating cuvettes are scanned by an integral spectrophotometer and the results displayed on an oscilloscope or relayed to a computer module for printout. One commercially available model (GEMSAEC, Electro-Nucleonics, Fairfield, New Jersey) has a capability of handling 300 samples per hour.

The difficulty with quantitative analytical procedures lies in the genetic interpretation of the results. Although any particular individual may consistently demonstrate for a given protein a very specific activity or quantity,[3] the population distribution of activities or quantities seldom has absolute discontinuities. This is not surprising, since the activity of a protein in a homeostatic organism is subject to a variety of regulatory mechanisms. The distribution of serum cholinesterase activity among homozygotes, e.g., is effectively continuous.[4] In the case of cholinesterase the 3 genotypes can be distinguished by differential inhibition of the catalytic activity of the enzyme with dibucaine. Such inhibition, however, reflects a specific qualitative difference between the "atypical" and normal proteins which would unlikely obtain in a randomly selected mutant of cholinesterase. Not only is there a wide spectrum of activity for the products of presumably identical alleles, but also a virtually continuous spectrum of activity for the products of different deficiency alleles as, for example, in the case of glucose-6-phosphate dehydrogenase.[5] The latter enzyme, incidentally, is especially amenable to analysis since a mutant allele can be examined in the hemizygous state. The detection of most rare variants, by quantitative means, would be complicated by the presence of a normal allele, varyingly active. A recently described rare electrophoretic variant of adenosine deaminase[6] with very little catalytic activity is one of many good examples of an activity variant which could not have been detected by quantitative techniques. The proportion of mutants which would lead to a change in the activity of a protein is unknown, although it must certainly vary

from locus to locus according to the structure of
the enzyme involved. The new efficiency in
quantitative analysis should prove exceedingly
useful in large scale screening for individuals
with a nearly complete loss of specific enzymatic activity (inborn errors of metabolism),
but an efficient ascertainment of new mutants
by these methods seems unlikely.

Variants separable from the type protein by
zone electrophoresis are inherited according to
simple mendelian rules[7] and in this respect are
eminently suitable for the detection of fresh
mutations. There is sufficient experience with
the inheritance of electrophoretic protein variants to suggest that under carefully controlled
conditions in some systems it will be safe to
assume that an electrophoretic variant in the
offspring of normal parents is genetically determined. This type of assumption is a requirement
for any reasonable monitoring system; if it were
necessary to establish by the inheritance pattern
in subsequent generations which variants among
the offspring of normal parents were mutants, one
could hardly monitor the human mutation rate for
the purpose of taking action to avoid a major
increase in new mutations.

Unfortunately, there is not at the moment an
efficient, inexpensive method for the large
scale screening of many proteins by electrophoresis. Existing manual procedures have been
improved somewhat by various minor alterations.
For example, in our own laboratory variants of
red cell adenylate kinase, 6-phosphogluconate
dehydrogenase, acid phosphatase phosphoglucomutase, adenosine deaminase, galactose-1
phosphate uridyl transferase and indophenol oxi-
dase have been detected in a single system
although the optimal length of time for electrophoresis does vary for different enzymes.[8] The

same conditions also resolve the isoenzymes of lactic dehydrogenase, malic dehydrogenase and phosphohexoseisomerase, and may well be useful for other enzymes. The gel can be sliced longitudinally, each slice being developed for several non-overlapping enzymes by the application of a mixture of the appropriate substrates, coenzymes and dyes. Good results are achieved using an agar overlay[9] but for a large scale program the expense of the reagents would be considerable. Fitch and Parr[10] have applied as little as one ml. of developing solution to an area of 150 cm[2] using a paint brush (compared to about 40 ml required in the agar method). In our hands better definition of the isoenzymes has been achieved by placing cellulose acetate strips soaked in 4 ml. of developing solution on top of the gel. These economies have been primarily directed toward the polymorphic enzymes, but presumably could also be applied to other systems in which enzyme variants have been resolved by electrophoresis. It should be possible without much difficulty to design a scheme whereby one technician could process 200 hemolysates for 15-20 enzymes per week. A similar efficiency is possible in the screening of serum proteins; we have, for example, detected variants of albumin, Group Specific Component, haptoglobin, transferrin and ceruloplasmin in a single electrophoretic system.[11]

The potential usefulness of electrophoresis in monitoring changes in the human germinal mutation rate depends on the answers to a number of questions. What proportion of mutants will result in variant proteins detectable by electrophoresis? What, then, is the estimated rate of detectable mutation? How important will the errors in labeling, handling, typing, and data processing be in relation to the expected inci-

dence of detectable mutant proteins? What is the
magnitude of the problem of the correct identification of the biological parents of a
suspected mutant? What will be the proportion
of actual mutants among the rare variants identified by screening? How many individuals must
be examined to effectively monitor a change in
the mutation rate, and how much technological
innovation will be required for reasonable
efficiency?

PROPORTION OF VARIANTS DETECTABLE
BY ELECTROPHORESIS

The data on hemoglobin mutants show no pre-
ponderance of transitions over transversions.[12]
Assuming this to be generally true, Kimura[13]
estimates the probability that a mutation would
result in no alteration of the amino acid
sequence at about 0.23. Approximately 25% of
the possible base changes in the allele for the
β-polypeptide chain of hemoglobin in this sense
are synonymous.[14] Of the remaining possible
mutations perhaps a third would result in the
substitution of an amino acid with a different
charge. For example, of the 2,217 amino acid
substitutions possible in the hemoglobin $\alpha\beta$ half
molecule on the basis of the genetic code, Sick
et al.[15] estimated that electrophoresis at pH 8.6
was potentially capable of detecting only 700
of these.

Smithies et al.[16] have demonstrated by the
recognition of additional allelic variability in
the α chain of haptoglobin following its separation from the β chain that not all charge differences may be recognizable in the intact protein.
The resolving power of electrophoresis, moreover,
depends very much on the specific conditions.
Shreffler et al.[17] examined 9000 Caucasian and

1000 Negro sera for ceruloplasmin without finding any variants. Yet by modifying their conditions only to the extent of diluting the sera
to 1/3 and changing electrophoresis from 16 hours
at 6v/cm to 22 hours at 7v/cm they were able to
detect variants with a frequency such that approximately 100 must have been missed in the
prior screening. The differential resolving
power of different electrophoretic systems has
been demonstrated for a number of proteins, and
it may be that no one system can be fully efficient in distinguishing different molecular
species.[18] Furthermore, systems which depend on
enzymatic activity can only detect variants
whose catalytic properties are not seriously
compromised. Identification of the position of
electrophoretically separated variants by a
precipitin reaction avoids the latter difficulty;
the method has potential[19] but has not had wide
application for this purpose, possibly because
of the labor involved in obtaining specific
antibodies. Current electrophoretic techniques
may in fact detect only 10% of allelic variability.

THE ESTIMATED RATE OF DETECTABLE MUTATION

From considerations of the energy of hydrogen
bonds, Watson[20] estimates that the average probability of an error in the insertion of a new
nucleotide during DNA replication under optimal
conditions may be 10^{-8} to 10^{-9}. Kimura[21] points
out that if the number of cell divisions along
the germ line from the fertilized egg to the
gamete is roughly 50, the rate of single base
mutation may be 5×10^{-7} to 5×10^{-8} per generation. Assuming the lower rate and assuming that
10% of mutations produce variants detectable in
a given electrophoretic system, the rate of

detectable mutations for a protein coded by 1000
nucleotide pairs may be 5×10^{-6} per protein
per generation. The estimate is not inconsistent
with an empirically determined spontaneous
forward mutation rate at five coat color loci
in the house mouse of 8.9×10^{-6} per locus per
gamete.[22] Assuming a rate per locus per generation of 10^{-5}, Crow[23] has pointed out that
virtually the entire annual population of new
births in the United States (3,000,000) would
have to be screened for new mutants at a given
locus in order to detect enough mutants (~60) to
determine a background mutation rate from which
it would be possible to establish an increase
of 1/3 in the incidence of new mutants as statistically significant. The number of individuals
screened could, of course, be reduced in proportion to the number of loci examined.

THE ERROR RATE

The large number of protein typings required
may pose a problem in relation to the probable
incidence of errors. For example, Sing et al.[24]
have typed 9182 Caucasians in 2507 two-genera-
tion families (1517 families in which both
parents were typed) for two serum proteins,
Secretor and red cell antigens in 8 systems.
Among the inconsistencies between parents and
offspring, 38 were determined to result from
labeling or data processing errors and 91 from
typing errors. These numbers are clearly under-
estimates since not all errors will result in
inconsistencies between parents and offspring.
My own experience with the electrophoresis of
perhaps 50,000 proteins suggests the error rate
for protein typing is unlikely to be much better.
An error rate of one per thousand, considering
the many steps involved between blood collection

and the entry of the correct genotype into a computer by manual techniques, would seem minimal even under favorable circumstances. The error rate exists in relation to a mutation rate 100 times less.

THE NONPATERNITY RATE

The identification of new mutants will assume that a child attributed to a given father and mother, and not clearly at variance genetically with them, is in fact their offspring. To evaluate the hazard of this assumption, it is necessary to know the incidence of nonpaternity and nonmaternity - that is, the situation in which the true parent is not correctly identified by historical information - and to know the probability of detecting the error on the basis of genetic information. Formulas for the estimation of the relationship between the over-all frequency of nonpaternity (α) and the frequency (D) with which it can be detected on the basis of examinations of mother, child and putative father have been developed.[25,26] Applied to a sample of 265 trios,[26] comprised wholly of Detroit Negroes which were examined with respect to the MN blood group system, the value for D is 0.038 and for α is 0.21 with a 95% confidence interval of 0.09 to 0.33. In their study of Caucasians in Tecumseh, Sing et al.[24] found that 3.76% of children had paternity exclusions and estimated that they had, by typing for 10 systems, detected 98% of the discrepancies. Given the low frequency of mutants and the high frequency of nonpaternity, the task of certifying, with a sufficiently high degree of probability, that an apparent mutant is indeed the child of a particular father appears, at face value, enormous.

THE PROPORTION OF NEW MUTANTS AMONG RARE VARIANTS

Any allele may be the result of a new mutation. The larger the proportion of variants
identified by screening which are examined with
respect to their inheritance the more complete
will be the ascertainment of new mutants. The
more common the variant, however, the less
likely it is the direct result of mutation.
Theoretically, one could type only the parents
of individuals possessing a variant which has a
limited frequency above the expected mutation
rate. Although any variant detected in a particular system is by definition distinguishable
from the type protein, it is not necessarily and
indeed unlikely to be distinguishable from all
other variants; information on the frequency of
specific rare variants simply does not exist.
The data for abnormal hemoglobins in Japan show
a frequency for all variants of about 0.0003.[27]
In screening 8000 Europeans, Sick et al.[15]
detected 11 hemoglobin variants, two of which
were identical and five of which had been previously unreported. A similar collective frequency of rare variants has been found for other
proteins in a number of surveys, generally of
1000-3000 individuals.[6,24, 28, 29, 30, 31] That
is, on the basis of the information available,
one can describe a class of variants which taken
together have a gene frequency less than 0.0005.
None of the 30 odd rare variants in the surveys
cited has been demonstrated to be the product
of a new mutant, often through more than one
generation. Considering only albumin variants
in populations in which the total variant gene
frequency is almost certainly less than 0.0005 [32]
we currently have studied 25 families, representing 11 electrophoretically distinguishable variants and in no instance have encountered any

evidence of a new mutation.[33] New mutants in man have been observed: Lehmann and Carrell[13] report receiving samples of Hb Hammersmith from two unrelated children, each of whose parents were unaffected - but they are clearly an uncommon finding among uncommon variants.

It is difficult to estimate the fraction of electrophoretically detectable mutants which will occur among those variants which as a class have a gene frequency less than 0.0005. Since there are relatively few polymorphic alleles in relation to the number of different mutants possible, this fraction will be significantly less than one only for those protein systems in which a particular electrophoretic technique cannot distinguish between a low frequency variant and the small variety of variants excluded from consideration as potential mutants by virtue of having a high frequency. If, for the purpose of speculation, this fraction is estimated to be 3/4, then the expected proportion of new mutants among the children with variants who are examined for the possibility of mutation will be 7.5 per thousand. A frequency of this magnitude does not pose an insuperable problem either with respect to errors in labeling, handling, typing and data processing or in terms of the assignment of the correct biological parents. If we ignore nonmaternity and assume an incidence of nonpaternity of, say, 6%, then on this basis 30 of 1000 children with variants will have two parents with the type allele. Thus, once the possibility of clerical and typing errors is eliminated, our a priori expectation is 4:1 in favor of nonpaternity over mutation as the correct explanation for the apparent biologic inconsistency. Under these conditions it should be possible in most cases to obtain statistically convincing evidence of the correct identification of the parents with the polymorphic marker systems currently available.

CONCLUSION

How many proteins in how many people must be screened? Assume that mutants detectable by current electrophoretic techniques occur at a rate of 5 x 10^{-6} per locus per generation. Assume that 1/4 of these will be missed by limiting the examination of families to those with children having variants rare enough to avoid major problems resulting from genotype inconsistencies due to sources other than mutation. Assume that only 2/3 of the families selected for investigation actually cooperate. Then 400,000 blood samples must be screened for 30 proteins to obtain enough variants to detect 60 mutants in perhaps 8000 families.

The major obstacle to the detection of electrophoretic protein variants as a method for monitoring the possibility of a change in the human germinal mutation rate is that in terms of current technology the task is formidable. While 15 scientists and 150 technicians with a budget of two million dollars might be able to accomplish it in a year, these resources do not exist, nor could such a large number of people be quickly mobilized. It can be anticipated that an increasing number of different and possibly more efficient methods will be applied to the search for variant proteins and that as a consequence the proportion of new mutants potentially detectable will increase. Current research projects, however, are insufficient to promote the development of an efficiency of the magnitude required for a mutation surveillance program. What is necessary is a concerted effort to design automatic techniques comparable in economy to those developed for quantitative analysis. Features which an electrophoretic surveillance system might include would be: 1) automatic sample withdrawal and application to a supporting medium; 2) conditions in which variants for a large number of proteins are separately recognizable in a single system; 3) recognition of the position of individual protein bands by a physical method which would be independent of biologic activity, rapid and quantitative; 4) conditions sufficiently reproducible that a computer can compare the pattern of protein bands to a series of type patterns and of this basis identify those individuals with rare variants; and 5) computer transfer of all phenotype information directly from the electrophoretic pattern to storage in final form.

The frequency of mutant proteins in the population is the most direct indicator of the germinal mutation rate available. Although an increased frequency of germinally determined mutant proteins is unlikely to yield a satisfactory clue to the identification of a mutagen, a specific knowledge of the germinal mutation rate may be useful in learning to interpret the results of a scheme more relevant in this respect as, perhaps, a somatic biochemical mutation monitoring system. There is in any event little doubt that rapid protein phenotyping would have many important genetic applications.

REFERENCES

1. Eckman I, Robbins JB, Van den Hamer CJA, et al: Automation of a quantitative immunochemical microanalysis of human serum transferrin: A model system. Clin Chem 16: 558-561, 1970
2. Anderson NG: The development of automated systems for clinical and research use. Clin Chim

Acta 25: 321-330, 1969

3. Hosenfeld D, Schröter E: Concerning the question of individual constancy and individual specificity of three serum enzyme activities (serum cholinesterase E C 3.1.1.8, ceruloplasmin E C 1.10.3.2, and alkaline phosphatase E C 3.1.3.1). Humangen 9: 38-42, 1970

4. Harris H, Whittaker M. Lehmann H, et al: The pseudocholinesterase variants. Esterase levels and dibucaine numbers in families selected through suxamethonium sensitive individuals. Acta Genet Stat Med 10: 1-16, 1960

5. Motulsky AG, Yoshida A: Methods for the study of red cell glucose-6-phosphate dehydrogenase, Biochemical Methods in Red Cell Genetics. Edited by JJ Yunis. New York, Academic Press, 1969, pp 51-93

6. Hopkinson DA, Cook PJL, Harris H: Further data on the adenosine deaminase (ADA) polymorphism and a report of a new phenotype. Ann Hum Genet (Lond) 32: 361-367, 1969

7. Harris H: Enzyme and protein polymorphisms in human populations. Brit Med Bull 25: 5-13, 1969

8. Weitkamp LR, Sing CF, Shreffler DC, et al: The genetic linkage relations of adenylate kinase: Further data on the ABO-AK linkage group. Amer J Hum Genet 21: 600-605, 1969

9. Fildes RA, Parr CW: Starch-gel electrophoresis of red-cell glucose-6-phosphate dehydrogenase. Biochem J 87: 45P, 1963

10. Fitch LI, Parr CW: Development of zymograms by the paintbrush technique. Biochem J 99: 20P, 1966

11. Weitkamp LR, Robson EB, Shreffler DC, et al: An unusual human serum albumin variant: Further data on genetic linkage between loci for human serum albumin and Group-Specific Component (Gc). Amer J Hum Genet 20: 392-397, 1968

12. Lehmann H, Carrell RW: Variations in the structure of human haemoglobin. Brit Med Bull 25: 14-23, 1969

13. Kimura M: Genetic variability maintained in a finite population due to mutational production of neutral and nearly neutral isoalleles. Genet Res (Camb) 11: 247-269, 1968

14. Harris H: The Principles of Human Biochemical Genetics. New York, American Elsevier Publishing Company, 1970

15. Sick K, Beale D, Irvine D et al: Haemoglobin G$_{Copenhagen}$ and Haemoglobin J$_{Cambridge}$. Two new -chain variants of haemoglobin A. Biochim Biophys Acta 140: 231-242, 1967

16. Smithies O, Connell GE, Dixon GH: Inheritance of haptoblobin subtypes. Am J Hum Genet 14: 14-21

17. Shreffler DC, Brewer GJ, Gall JC, et al: Electrophoretic variation in human serum ceruloplasmin: A new genetic polymorphism. Biochem Genet 1: 101-115, 1967

18. Weitkamp, LR, Franglen G, Rokala DA, et al: An electrophoretic comparison of human serum albumin variants: Eight distinguishable types. Hum Hered 19: 159-169, 1969

19. Szeinberg A, Zoreff E, Golan R: Immunoelectrophoretic-chemical investigation of erythrocyte aspartate aminotransferase. Life Sci 8: 943-948, 1969.

20. Watson, JD: Molecular Biology of the Gene. New York, WA Benjamin, 1965

21. Kimura M: Evolutionary rate at the molecular level. Nature 217: 624-626, 1968

22. Schlager G, Dickie MM: Spontaneous mutations and mutation rates in the house mouse. Genet 57: 319-330, 1967

23. Crow JF: Human population monitoring, environmental Chemical Mutagens. Edited by A Hollaender, Plenum Press, in press

24. Sing CF, Shreffler DC, Neel JV, et al: Studies on genetic selection in a completely ascertained Caucasian population. II. Family analysis of eleven blood group systems. Amer J Hum Genet, in press

25. MacCluer JW, Schull WJ: On the estimation of the frequency of nonpaternity. Amer J Hum Genet 15: 191-202, 1963

26. Potthoff RF, Whittinghill M: Maximum likelihood estimation of the proportion of nonpaternity. Amer J Hum Genet 17: 480-494, 1965

27. Livingston FB: Abnormal Hemoglobins in Human Populations. Chicago, Aldine Publishing Company, 1967

28. Hopkinson DA, Harris H: Rare phosphoglucomutase phenotypes. Ann Hum Genet (Lond) 30: 167-181, 1966

29. Lewis WHP, Harris H: Human red cell peptidase. Nature 215: 351-355, 1967

30. Detter JC, Ways PO, Giblett ER, et al: Inherited variations in human phosphohexoseisomerase. Ann Hum Genet (Lond) 31: 329-338, 1968

31. Weitkamp LR, Neel JV: Gene frequencies and microdifferentiation among the Makiritare Indians. III. Nine erythrocyte enzyme systems. Am J Hum Genet 22: 533-537, 1970

32. Cooke KB, Cleghorn TE, Lockey E: Two new families with bisalbuminemia: An examination of possible links with other genetically controlled variants. Biochem J 81: 39P-40P, 1961

33. Weitkamp LR, Renwick JH, Berger J: Additional data and summary for albumin-Gc linkage in man. Hum Hered 20: 1-7, 1970

COMMENTS ON BIOCHEMICAL MONITORING

H. Eldon Sutton

It is important to recognize that the preceding two papers deal with screening for two types of phenomena, for which there are at least two objectives. Dr. Scheinberg's concern with the detection of variant alleles is directed toward the detection of individuals who have disease due to genetic causes, rather than with the mutation process. Monitoring in this sense, then, is a matter of bringing medical care to the public. This program should probably be part of the routine examination of young children as it is important to identify disease as early as possible, especially if treatment is available.

On the other hand, Dr. Weitkamp's interest and that of several others here lies with the detection of mutations as a genetic process. Their objective in monitoring is to recognize environmental changes which are altering the genetic constitution, regardless of whether the change evokes disease. Although we know that this kind of mutation is also producing mutant genes which do cause disease, we are concentrating here on systems which give us information on the process, not necessarily on the diseases which may be produced at the same time.

This difference in objective is related to the kinds of systems observed. It is important for Dr. Scheinberg's objectives to examine the systems which are directly concerned with disease.

Most of the major genetic diseases are disorders related to the loss of function of some particular protein, e.g., an enzyme function. The variant genes which remain functional are not of concern in this system. There are many polymorphic systems where several alleles appear to behave normally; these are of no interest in disease. They may have other genetic interests, but not in this particular system. The techniques of screening with this kind of objective should reflect the function which the protein carries out for normal development, such as the presence or absence of enzyme activity. These functional variants might be missed if their detection depended upon qualitative data such as protein sequence, electrophoretic patterns and immunologic reactions.

The requirements for screening for mutations are somewhat different. Here we are interested in whether the protein represents a new mutation, not in whether the protein is functional. In addition to the requirements summarized for such systems by Dr. Weitkamp, there is one that has to do with dominant versus recessive effects. In practice, it is not very useful to look for a mutant gene that is expressed recessively. It's difficult to identify and since the recessive disorders are extremely sensitive to inbreeding, and to small differences in fitness of heterozygotes, they have not yet yielded useful information on mutation rates. One must look for dominant expressions of a mutant gene for information on mutation rates, therefore, and this rather limits us to protein property changes, such as electrophoresis, which reflect a change in the primary structure of the protein.

I should like to underscore one of Dr. Weitkamp's requirements, that one should look for rare variants. This is a practical matter.

A change in the mutation rate of variant hemoglobins, for example, would be more easily
detected in a Caucasian population where they
are rare, than in Negroes where the frequency of
Hemoglobin S is so high that it would not be a
useful index of the mutation rate. So, one is
limited here to the exotic variant and must
avoid the polymorphic variants or those classified with polymorphisms.

The two types of studies may well overlap, and
rightly so, in the collection of samples which
is a considerable part of large scale studies.
There is no reason why a single collection
system would not profitably serve the two
objectives.

PROSPECTS OF MONITORING ENVIRONMENTAL MUTAGENESIS THROUGH SOMATIC MUTATIONS

H. Eldon Sutton

Somatic mutations have an extensive history of involvement in genetic theory, but they have had limited opportunity for study, especially in higher animals. Somatic mutations have been invoked to explain aging, cancer, and immune processes in man. Yet, only one class of somatic mutations, chromosome aberrations, has been the subject of systematic investigation. Point mutations affecting only a single gene or chromosome deletions too small to be visible are completely unexplored. Indeed, they have often been considered to be rather exotic events, important perhaps but not amenable to study.

One stumbling block has been the traditional definition of mutation -- a heritable change. In the case of germinal mutations at

*

The studies reported from this laboratory have been supported in part by U.S. Public Health Service Contract 70-228, grant GM 09326, and Career Development Award E K03 GM 18,381.

least those which do not confer sterility, transmission of a newly appearing trait to subsequent generations is strong evidence of genetic mutation, especially if the transmission obeys Mendel's laws. But there are no Mendelian laws for somatic transmission, and a newly arising variation limited to somatic cells of an individual could be due to processes other than mutation. One must interpret somatic variation with great care and be conservative in attributing it to mutation.

The time has come however when a major effort must be put into detecting somatic mutations. The impetus for this is the concern for the mutagenic effects of environmental agents. If such agents do influence the rate of somatic mutations, and thereby the rate of aging and of carcinogenesis, it is important to identify these effects and to identify the responsible agents. Furthermore, it is a safe assumption that agents which cause somatic mutations also cause germinal mutations, giving rise to defective children in subsequent generations. In somatic mutations, the damage dies with the individual.

At present, there is no information relating somatic and germinal mutation rates, and there are substantial theoretical difficulties in transferring results from one tissue to another. Without attempting a thorough review or analysis, I will mention one problem. Germinal mutation rates are conveniently expressed as mutations/locus/generation (or per gamete). This implies that the origins of germinal mutations are somehow primarily related to life cycles. But a life cycle is composed of many cell cycles, the number depending on the tissue. Further, in the germ line, there is a large difference in the number of cycles in human females and males. Would mutation rates be more meaningful in terms of cell cycles as compared to life cycles, or would a denominator of absolute time be more useful? The answer will come only with observations yet to be made.

While somatic mutation has been evoked to explain a variety of observations, the only systematic investigations in man appear to be those of Atwood (1958) and Atwood and Scheinberg (1959). These authors devised techniques for measuring the proportion of red cells lacking an antigen inherited by the donor and present in the majority of cells. They found that persons of blood type A who are genetically heterozygous for A and O have a small portion of cells, usually about 0.1%, which do not react with antisera to A. Further, Atwood (1958) showed that cells which do not express the inherited A_1 antigen may express the genetically alternate A_2 properties. In later studies, the proportions of variant cells were not found to conform to simple expectations based on a hypothesis of somatic mutation (Atwood and Pepper, 1961). More complex interactions were not ruled out, and the important test of transmissibility is not available for erythrocytes.

These studies and others provide clear evidence for the existence of variant cells which do not express the predominant genotype of the person and which have not been explained as part of the normal differentiation process. Possibly they are mutant cells with altered genetic information. As yet there has been no demonstration that the genetic information is altered--or more practically, that the variation is transmissible. Possibly somatic crossing over and selection, separately or together, cause major deviation from the mutational models with which the results have been compared.

Is it possible to devise a system for detecting and quantifying somatic mutations in spite of these difficulties? I believe that the answer is yes. It has become commonplace to study the phenotypes of individual cells using sensitive biochemical methods. Conventionally, cytology has focused on the mass cell phenotype rather than the scarce phenotype. This, of course, is appropriate for the kinds of questions which have been asked. But, I believe that some additional answers can be obtained if new questions are asked.

For purposes of argument, let us assume that the same kinds of mutations can occur somatically that are known to occur germinally. This would include a wide array of base pair substitutions, leading to amino acid substitutions in proteins, as well as deletions or other rearrangements of information, often leading to absence of a specific polypeptide chain. These mutations are assumed to occur at frequencies characteristic of the specific mutation and dependent on a variety of environmental agents, as well as the inherited metabolic environment of the cell. Even though the mutations are very rare, they would tend to accumulate unless they conferred a selective disadvantage on the cell. If methods can be devised which are sufficiently sensitive to identify individual mutant cells in the midst of a mass of nonmutant cells, it should be possible to assess the cumulative mutational risk of a person at any point in his life.

The assumptions and contingencies are large but not necessarily insurmountable. The life span of man is long by microbial standards but the generation time of cells in certain tissues is very short. For example, the generation time of the stem cells of the blood

forming elements appears to be on the order of
one and a half to two days. The stem cells of a
middle aged person might thus have gone through
ten thousand replications since conception.
Whatever the mutation rate per cell cycle, it
could be multiplied by 10^4 to obtain the accum-
mulated mutations. A value of 10^{-7} for a
specific amino acid substitution might thus have
accumulated to a frequency on the order of one
mutant gene per thousand. Even if this value is
an order of magnitude too high, it might still
be possible to devise screening methods for
counting accurately the variant cells. Furthermore, many of the methods devised would undoubtedly sum together several mutations which share
the variant phenotype even though the structural
causes might differ.

An effective means of detecting and monitoring somatic mutations depends on developing
systems in which the variant cells react positively compared to nonvariant cells, with good
discrimination between positive and negative
cells. Many mutations are known which reduce
or destroy enzymatic activity. A negative cell
in a mass of positive cells may be identifiable,
but the reasons for failure of a reaction are
many, and interpretation of rare negative cells
will always be suspect. This unfortunately
rules out most of the known genetic variants of
enzymes.

Ideally, variants should be observed in
easily accessible tissue, such as blood cells.
For meaningful interpretation, mutant cells
should have no selective advantage or disadvantage. Further, there should be no or few phenocopies. To be maximally useful in a monitoring
system, mutant cells should be identifiable by
automated methods, although this is not an
absolute necessity.

One system explored in my laboratory may
serve as a candidate for a monitoring system for
somatic mutations. The enzyme glucose-6-phos-
phate dehydrogenase occurs in many inherited
variant forms (World Health Organization, 1967).
One recent estimate is that greater than 70
forms are known, but identity has not been dis-
proved for all combinations of variants. Many
of the variants have been studied in detail with
regard to kinetic properties. Most have a
broadened pH range. Two rare variants, Gd
Markham (Kirkman et al., 1968) and Gd Union
(Yoshida et al.,1970) are noteworthy because
of their greatly broadened substrate specificity
as well as pH range. The usual enzyme acts only
with NADP as cofactor and acts only upon glucose-
6-phosphate as substrate, converting it to
6-phosphogluconate. There is a single peak in
the pH activity curve. Gd Markham and Gd Union
both act on 2-deoxy-glucose-6-phosphate as substrate, reacting even faster than with glucose-
6-phosphate. They also will act on galactose-6-
phosphate, and Gd Markham will use NAD as
cofactor. These are examples of minor alterations in the structure of the protein portion
of an enzyme resulting in general loss of
reaction specificity. The enzyme becomes compatible with a greater variety of molecules.

The effect of such decreased specificity is to
confer new enzymatic activities on the variant
molecule. It should be possible to detect cells
carrying variant forms of the enzyme by their
ability to react with artificial substrates
when nonvariant cells will not. We thus have met
a requirement given earlier which is technically
very important: the variant cells give positive
reactions.

Attempts to apply this theory to real cells
have been successful so far as detecting variant

cells is concerned. Methods had already been developed for detection of glucose-6-phosphate dehydrogenase in individual cells. Briefly, the method consists in detecting reduced NADP produced during the enzymatic reaction. NADPH will react with various tetrazolium dyes to produce an insoluble precipitate in the presence of phenazine. We adapted these procedures to white blood cells. With glucose-6-phosphate as substrate, most of the cells become filled with dark precipitate, reacting strongly positive. With 2-deoxyglucose-6-phosphate, most cells are completely negative, a few rare cells are slightly positive, and a few more are strongly positive (Figure 1).

The frequency of strongly positive cells is approximately 0.001. This value is remarkably close to expectation for mutant cells as proposed earlier, but that may be entirely coincidence. Most of our effort has been concentrated on improving the techniques of observation. We now have enough data to suggest individual differences in the frequencies of variant cells, although the period of observation is short. If these variant cells are mutants, there should be an age correlation. Inspection of the limited data does not suggest a correlation, but this may mean that other factors are much more important.

Before we can propose this particular system as detecting mutant cells, it will be necessary to demonstrate that the variant phenotypes are transmitted to daughter cells. Since the variants are found among lymphocytes, this task is potentially soluble, although we have not succeeded as yet. Other approaches would be to show that the variants are increased by known mutagenic agents, although interpretation in this case would be subject to some argument.

The important point of these studies is the demonstration that phenotyping of individual cells is possible. With sufficient effort, systems can be found which will identify mutant cells. If enough such systems are found, the mutational experiences of a person can be assessed accurately. With proper epidemiological consideration, it should be possible to identify some of the factors, environmental or otherwise, which increase somatic mutation.

Albertini and DeMars (1970) have published studies showing the isolation of fibroblasts mutant for hypoxanthine-guanine phosphoribosyl transferase (HGPRT) from cultures of cells with normal HGPRT. This enzyme is responsible for conversion of hypoxanthine to inosine 5'-monophosphate and of guanine to guanosine 5'-monophosphate. The structure of the enzyme is determined by a gene on the X chromosome. Mutants of this enzyme are known in man, the resulting deficiency of activity causing Lesch-Nyhan syndrome, a condition in which there is elevated plasma uric acid and severe mental deficiency resulting in self mutilation.

The system of Albertini and DeMars utilized the conversion of 8-azaguanine to its nucleotide by cells with normal HGPRT, leading to inhibition of growth. Cells mutant for HGPRT cannot convert 8-azaguanine to the corresponding nucleotide and, therefore, are quite resistant to inhibition. By incorporating 8-azaguanine into culture medium inoculated with normal cells, only mutants deficient for HGPRT can grow. These authors isolated two such mutants from two different cell lines, demonstrating the feasibility of using specific human loci to test for mutation.

The HGPRT system has the advantage of being

readily adaptable to testing of specific compounds for mutagenicity. In this, it comple-
ments the microbial systems already in use. To
be adapted for monitoring of human populations,
it will be necessary to devise a means of samp-
ling tissues without intervening in vitro
culture. This may be of questionable practicality for fibroblasts. If the systems for cloning
lymphocytes, such as that reported by Dr. Bloom,
can be developed for large scale observations,
it should be possible to devise a means of
detecting mutations pre-existing in the body.

An entirely different system for studying
somatic mutation has been suggested by recent
demonstrations that unscheduled DNA synthesis
occurs in vivo in epidermal layers of human
skin (e.g. Epstein et al., 1970). Ultraviolet
radiation causes formation of thymine dimers in
DNA. In E. coli and in man there exist repair
mechanisms whereby such dimers are excised by an
endonuclease, the proper bases are inserted, and
the complete double-stranded DNA is restored.
The incorporation of radioactively labeled
thymine into DNA during a period when DNA replication is not scheduled is a measure of repair
of recent DNA lesions. Patients with xeroderma
pigmentosum are defective in the repair process
(Cleaver, 1969).

Study of this system up to now has been
largely concerned with ultraviolet-induced
alterations of DNA. The system is more general,
however, and it possibly may be adapted to other
mutagens. Such a procedure would reflect recent
mutation only. It might be especially useful
therefore, in recognizing mutation after
exposure to specific agents. Such a system
would be helpful in identifying which of the
myriad of environmental experiences is important
in mutation.

I will not attempt to discuss somatic chromosomal aberrations, since they are considered by other speakers. The distinction between chromosomal aberrations and point mutations is primarily operational and there is substantial overlap in causes. On the other hand, there is some specificity of mutagenic agents and resultant mutations. This is especially so comparing point mutations to chromosomal aberrations, but it is also true comparing certain point mutations to other aberrations. Thus, monitoring by several systems, including both chromosomal and point mutations, yields information not available in any one system.

This brief discussion of possibilities for quantitative studies of somatic mutation in man is a bit heavy on theory and light on accomplishment. It is intended to help identify directions in which research may prove beneficial. Monitoring for somatic chromosome aberrations is being done now by several laboratories, none on a large-scale systematic basis. More funds could permit large scale monitoring with existing technology, although whether this is the best use of funds and whether greater automation should be introduced first are questions I shall not attempt to answer. I also believe that methods of detecting somatic biochemical mutations can be readily developed based largely on existing knowledge.

It is possible, perhaps probable, that none of the methods discussed today will be in use ten years from now. I hope that this is because better methods and new ideas will make them obsolete.

REFERENCES

Albertini, R. J. and DeMars, R., 1970.

Diploid azaguanine-resistant mutants of cultured human fibroblasts. Science 169: 482-485.

Atwood, K.C., 1958. The presence of A2 erythrocytes in A1 blood. Proc. Nat. Acad.Sci. (U.S.) 44: 1054-1057.

Atwood, K.C., and Pepper, F.J. 1961. Erythrocyte automosaicism in some persons of known genotype. Science 134: 2100-2102.

Atwood, K.C., and Scheinberg, S.L. 1959. Isotope dilution method for assay of inagglutinable erythrocytes. Science 129: 963-964.

Cleaver, J.E. 1969. Xeroderma pigmentosum: a human disease in which an initial stage of DNA repair is defective. Proc. Nat. Acad.Sci. (U.S.) 63: 428-435.

Epstein, J.H., Fukuyama, K., Reed, W.B., and Epstein, W.L. 1970. Defect in DNA synthesis in skin of patients with xeroderma pigmentosum demonstrated in vivo. Science 168: 1477-1478.

Kirkman, H.N., Kidson, C., and Kennedy, M., 1968. Variants of human glucose-6-phosphate dehydrogenase. Studies of samples from New Guinea. In Beutler, E. (ed.), Hereditary Disorders of Erythrocyte Metabolism. Grune and Stratton, New York, pp. 126-140.

World Health Organization. 1967. Nomenclature of glucose-6-phosphate dehydrogenase in man. Bull. WHO 36: 319-322. Reprinted in Amer. J. Human Genet. 19: 757-761 (1967).

Yoshida, A., Baur, E.W., and Motulsky, A.G. 1970. A Philippino glucose-6-phosphate dehydrogenase variant (G6PD Union) with enzyme deficiency and altered substrate specificity. Blood 35: 506-513.

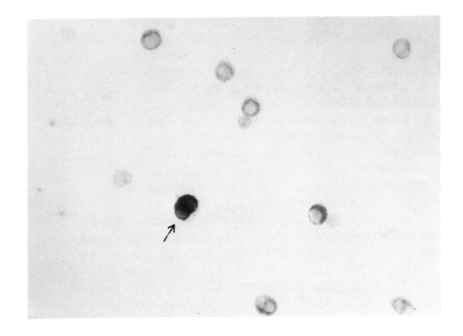

Figure 1. A white blood cell preparation showing activity of one cell (indicated by arrow) with 2-deoxyglucose-6-phosphate as substrate. Cells were suspended in a reaction mixture which was 0.15 M NaCl, 0.4 M Tris (pH 9.1), and 0.006 M 2-deoxyglucose-6-phosphate; and contained 0.4 mg. NADP, 6-7 units streptodornase, 0.26 mg. nitro blue tetrazolium, and 0.06 mg phenazine methosulfate per ml. After one hour at 30°C, the cells are washed with buffered saline and a suspension of cells is spread on a cover slip. The cells are dried thoroughly and are counterstained with neutral red. Positive cells are dark purple or are densely packed with dark granules. Negative cells are red.

MONITORING FOR CHROMOSOMAL ABNORMALITY IN MAN*

Maimon M. Cohen
Arthur D. Bloom

INTRODUCTION

The suggested programs of monitoring human populations for mutagenesis have been based largely on three approaches: the detection of phenotypic deviation -- the appearance of an inordinate increase in various mutant, or sentinel, phenotypes; the detection of biochemical polymorphisms -- qualitative alterations in serum or cellular proteins or enzymes; and the detection of cytogenetic abnormality -- either numerical or structural.[1] Of these three possibilities, the consensus, at this point in time, seems to favor cytogenetic investigation as the most practicable method, because of the currently available technology and the imminent possibility of applying automated techniques to population screening. At present, the two other procedures are yet impractical on a

---

*

Supported in part by a grant (to M.M.C.) from the U.S. Children's Bureau (Project No. 417) and by grants (to A.D.B.) from the National Institute of General Medical Sciences (NIH-1-P01-GM-15419-04) and the Atomic Energy Commission AT(11-1)-1552.

population level.

The use of cytogenetic screening has for many years been interpreted as a useful indicator of environmental effects on genetic material. Those postulates concerning mutagenesis derived from studies on the chromosome systems of lower organisms (e.g., plants and drosophila), have been borne out for the most part by mammalian and, more recently, human cytogenetics.

The chromosomal abnormalities most easily detected are those of number and structure. Numerical abnormalities have been ascertained almost exclusively through phenotypic deviation, with a rather impressive correlation between karyotype and phenotype (e.g., trisomies 13, 18, 21; Turner's Syndrome; and Klinefelter's Syndrome). While the association between structural abnormalities (which involve chromosome breakage) and phenotype might be obvious in some cases (e.g., the Cri-du-Chat Syndrome), in the vast majority of cases, the phenotype is extremely variable and too nonspecific to be useful as an indicator of chromosomal abnormality. Therefore, direct cytological observation is needed.

More important perhaps is the phenomenon of chromosome breakage which does not result in a single structural anomaly, but in a generalized increase in chromosome damage in somatic cells. Although such chromosome damage may be a useful parameter of environmental hazards, the significance of these aberrations is at best poorly understood.

MECHANISMS OF CHROMOSOME BREAKAGE

A variety of agents are capable of producing cellular effects which become manifest as chromosome damage. These include ionizing radiations, viruses, and various chemicals. The chemicals

can be subdivided into those compounds affecting
the biosynthesis of informational macromolecules
(DNA, RNA and protein); anti-tumor agents; antibiotics; mono-and bifunctional alkylating agents;
nitroso-compounds and an ill-defined heterogeneous group of compounds.[2-7] It should be
emphasized that it is not necessarily the chromosomal breaks per se, but the mechanisms by which
they arise, which are of greatest interest.
These mechanisms will ultimately yield important
information concerning chromosome structure and
function. Although chromosome breaks may morpho-
logically appear identical, and their distribution along the chromosome similar, independent of
the inducing agent,[6] it is highly probable that
the various agents act through quite dissimilar
mechanisms.

The postulate mechanisms underlying chemically
induced chromosome breakage are many and varied,
but can be divided into several general categories. These include direct involvement of DNA
(either pre-or post-synthesis) through inhibition, degradation or impairment of template
activity; alkylation; lack of repair; and, enzymatic digestion of chromosomes. (For detailed
discussion of mechanisms of chromosome breakage,
see Kihlman[4] and Cohen, Hirschhorn and Freeman.[8])

CORRELATION OF CHROMOSOME DAMAGE WITH MUTAGENESIS

The essence of any population monitoring program, from a genetic viewpoint, is to utilize
parameters which discriminate genetic change or
mutation. Chromosome abnormality in and of itself does not suggest mutation. Although phenotypic deviation is invariably associated with
gross alteration in chromosome number, chromosome
damage (breakage) may indicate a more insidious,

subtle, and sometimes subobservational genetic alteration. If the effect is extreme, cell death will most likely follow. However, the more important considerations, from a population basis, are those effects which allow for cell survival in the presence of more or less balanced chromosome rearrangements which are capable of being transmitted (e.g., translocations, insertions, pericentric inversions).

While the production of chromosome breakage is not necessarily a measure of point mutations, extensive circumstantial evidence exists which links chromosomal abnormalities and mutation. Radiation studies clearly yield increases in both chromosome breakage and mutations. Additionally, studies of chemicals generally support this association. Comparison of various chemicals known to induce chromosomal damage in plant and mammalian cells have also demonstrated mutagenesis in other systems.[6] Likewise, agents known to be mutagenic in test systems specifically designed to detect such phenomena (e.g., the dominant lethal test[9] or the host mediated assay[10]) have almost invariably been found to produce chromosomal damage. Therefore, even though chromosomal damage may not directly prove that an agent is mutagenic, the association between mutagenesis and chromosome damage is by no means an uncommon occurrence. Thus, while screening for chromosomal damage may provide a rapid and sensitive method for studying the cellular effects of environmental agents, it should be coupled with other test systems which are specifically designed to detect mutagenic effects in microorganisms or experimental animals.

METHODS OF MONITORING FOR CHROMOSOME DAMAGE

Cytogenetic screening depends on the detection

of microscopically visible chromosome changes.
Those changes involving chromosome breakage often
lead to frank loss or exchange of genetic material. In addition to breakage, gain or loss of
entire chromosomes (nondisjunction) or sets of
chromosomes (polyploidy) are sometimes seen.
Experiments are easily constructed which will
yield quantitative information relative to possible mutagens and the genetic apparatus. Some
of the easiest and most approachable questions
are those concerned with the effects on the
mitotic index; the time of action of an agent in
the cell cycle; correlation of chromosome damage
with concentration and duration of exposure; the
types of damage induced; and the possible non-
random localization of damage to specific regions
of chromosomes.

The methodologies necessary for the study of
chromosomal aberrations are already well developed and widely applied. These techniques require a population of dividing cells, or a population that is induced to divide through some
external mitogenic stimulus. The accumulation of
metaphase cells with agents such as colchicine is
usually employed, but is not absolutely necessary.
A number of efficient methods are available for
adequate preparation of cells for microscopic
observation. (For a detailed description of
methods of cell preparation for chromosome analysis, see Cohen and Hirschhorn.[11])

These cytogenetic techniques may be used in the
study of the somatic and germinal tissues of a
wide choice of experimental animals as well as
man. Further, both in vitro and in vivo cytogenetic examinations may be performed. Additionally,
the development of amniocentesis for chromosome
evaluation adds yet another dimension to the
flexibility of this approach -- that of antenatal
detection and the prevention of the appearance of

chromosomally abnormal individuals, particularly in high risk pregnancies.

To date, short term cultures of circulating leukocytes offer, perhaps, the most valuable tool for studies of the experimental induction of karyotypic defects and for the possible monitoring of human populations. The use of chromosomal damage as a dosimeter after acute radiation exposure is well established.[12-14] Perhaps, similar approaches may be used to study individuals who have undergone long-term exposure to chemicals. The short-term leukocyte culture technique provides a ready access to cells that were exposed in vivo and allows repeated samplings with little hazard or inconvenience to the subject. Only minute amounts of blood are needed and such studies may be performed on humans as well as extended to many animal species.

SCORING OF CHROMOSOME ABNORMALITIES

Any classification of chromosomal effects combines terminologies from morphological descriptions and the physiologic processes from which they derive. The actual scoring of chromosomal abnormalities may be done according to various systems of nomenclature.[15-19] In practice, there are three possible consequences of chromosome breakage: 1) Chromatid aberrations; 2) Chromosome aberrations; 3) Restitution, which occurs in most cases. To differentiate between some of the morphological forms arising from chromatid and chromosome type aberrations is often difficult in metaphase cells. Obvious differences, however, may be clearly seen in anaphase figures (for discussion, see Kihlman). From a practical point of view, however, in metaphase plates, two types of chromosomal damage can be observed--simple chromosome breaks and complex structural rearrangements. The importance of structural rearrangements derives from the fact that most morphologic aberrations arise through the exchange of chromatid fragments between two chromosomes. A number of agents cause simple breaks which are mitotically unstable and those cells carrying such abnormalities tend to disappear rapidly from the circulation. However, radiation, radiomimetic drugs, oncogenic viruses, and diseases associated with a high incidence of leukemia (e.g., Fanconi's anemia and Bloom's syndrome) are all associated with structural rearrangements, including translocations, leading to mitotically stable chromosomal aberrations[20] which may proliferate in vivo to form clones of abnormal cells.

Abnormalities are usually scored as breaks only if a clear discontinuity of the chromatid is visible and if nonalignment of the chromatid axis is obvious. Breaks are classified as "chromatid" if only a single chromatid is affected and "isochromatid" if both sister chromatids are broken at the same location. Single chromatid fragments are usually included with chromatid breaks while "double fragments" are considered, in most cases, to be the result of only a single break, though they may be the result of two breaks in a G_2 cell where the chromosome is duplicated. The structural rearrangements which can be assessed are usually the result of two or more breaks. Ring chromosomes, dicentric chromosomes and obvious translocations are examples of "two-hit' phenomena. Complex rearrangements leading to abnormal morphological forms such as triradials, quadriradials and pulverized nuclei result from multiple breaks. Attenuated pale staining regions, other than the secondary contrictions described as normal in the human karyotype[21],[22] which do not show obvious nonalignment, are usually scored as "gaps" and are generally not included in the calculation of breakage rates.

The sole criterion for the designation of anomalies as chromatid or isochromatid breaks has been the principle of nonalignment of the chromatid axis. However, recent work, utilizing both electron microscopy and phase contrast microscopy of the same metaphase cell, has indicated that perhaps this requirement of nonalignment may not be the optimal discriminant. Aberrations which in phase contrast appeared as achromatic, aligned gaps were observed in the electron microscope as clean breaks. Conversely, some breaks which were obviously nonaligned, with a considerable separation of the distal fragment from the remainder of the chromatid, showed obvious microfibrils stretching between the two segments.[23]

TECHNICAL CONSIDERATIONS

Control cells for in vitro studies should be obtained from the same donor(s) if exogenous agents are to be added to cultures. If in vivo effects are being tested, it is preferable to study cells of the same subject sequentially, i.e., before and after drug administration. Control and treated individuals should be matched as closely as possible for obvious factors such as sex, age, race and occupation. Cultures should, of course, be propagated and processed in parallel, utilizing the same lots of medium, trypsin, colcemide, fixative and stains, and should be manipulated on the same day. Because of the possibility of near-toxic effects of chemicals, or of unwanted viruses, upon chromosome morphology and on entry of cells into mitosis, it may be useful to add a known chromosome breaking agent, as a positive control.

Valid comparisons of data depend on internal consistency in method during microscopic examination, that is, fixed criteria for the kinds of aberrations scored. Reliable cytological scoring demands equal attention to each cell examined and to each parameter considered. This is necessary in the face of problems of observer fatigue and possible observer bias. Ideally, cultures should be randomized and referred to only by coded numbers assigned by others. Even in the same material, truly comparable opportunities for detection of chromosome aberrations obtain only in metaphase cells which are similar in degrees of condensation and in cytological quality. For reasons not understood, chromosome preparations from bone marrow cells are generally of poorer cytological quality than those from cultured fibroblasts or leukocytes; but, in general, these differences are not limiting. Variation in quality necessitates the selection of usable metaphases, a selection usually made under low power optics.

The time necessary for careful microscopic analysis is considerable and, therefore, many studies published are simply inadequate in terms of the numbers of cells examined. Unwarranted extrapolations of the findings beyond a few subjects should be avoided and statistical handling of the observed variability must utilize the appropriate tests for differences between means[24,25] or for variances between two populations[26] or for small samples.[27]

AUTOMATION OF CHROMOSOMAL SCREENING

With the above limitations in mind and with greater demands being made for large scale screening procedures, it becomes obvious that manual methods of chromosome analysis are inadequate. Therefore, methods are currently being devised for the automation of cytogenetic analysis. These methods, at present, are in the developmental stage and provide a series of diverse approaches to the solution of the problem. Some techniques are semi-automated while others are completely so. However, the goal of all such systems is the rapid screening of large numbers of cells which will make population monitoring a practicality. Such systems will yield quantitative information which can be utilized to define, more stringently, the normal human karyotype and subtle variations thereof, as well as to aid in studies of chromosomal mutagenesis.

Each of the systems presently under development consists of four basic components: 1) Location of suitable metaphase cells: 2) Scanning of the input image (either directly or from photographic prints or negatives) and the conversion of such visual data to computer information; 3) Computer analysis of input data and generation of karyotypes; and 4) Statistical analysis of the resultant data. Each of these parts of the system may be completely automated or sometimes semi-automated, or may have to remain manual, depending on the individual system used. For example, one method devised by Lubs and Ruddle[28] is considered to be semi-automated. The completely computerized steps are those dealing with data storage, karyotype construction and data analysis. The location of cells and obtaining of an input image (in this case photographic negatives) remains completely manual. The actual measurement is done with a semi-automated XY digitizer which records the X and Y coordinates of the various chromosome landmarks (e.g., centromere, end of arm, satellites, secondary constrictions). These data are then recorded on magnetic tape and recalculated by a high speed digital computer. In final form, the chromosomes are grouped according to length and arm ratio. An experienced operator can analyze a single cell in 20 minutes at a cost of approximately $3 to $5 per cell. A similar semi-automated system has been described by Bender and Kastenbaum[29] using a pair of dividers, one point of which is placed at the centromere of the chromosome and the other point at the end of the arm. The measurements for each chromosome thus consist of a set of four, two for the short arm and two for the long arm. The data so obtained are punched on cards and analyzed by computer.

The ultimate goal, however, is obviously the development of completely automated systems which eliminate the necessity for human intervention, except in a supervisory capacity. Several different approaches to this problem have been tried, but we will only discuss one of them as a model for the others. The methods for data storage, retrieval and analysis by computer techniques have been devised by people in fields other than cytogenetics. Perhaps, the greatest problem we face, from the standpoint of consumption of investigators' time and necessitating human value judgements, is the selection of the proper cell for analysis. Most automated systems rely on input data (photographic prints or negatives) already supplied, but Wald et al.[30] are developing an automated microscope which is capable of screening slides and discriminating metaphase cells from other "noise" objects on the slide such as stain particles and bubbles. Microscope

slides are prepared by routine techniques and
hand loaded onto a revolving stage, six at a time.
The stage rotates at approximately 20 RPM and the
slides pass through the first of two light
sources--a laser beam. The beam scatter is analyzed through photomultipliers, for patterns dis-
cernible as metaphase plates. When a decision is
made that a suitable object has been located, its
slide position is recorded automatically. Each
recorded position is then relocated and analyzed
with a high resolution optical system. After
automatic focusing, the cell is scanned by a
"flying spot" scanner and the image is converted
to binary form for computer processing. In this
system, the cytological material itself is used
with no intermediary step of photographic prints
or negatives being necessary. The practicality
of this system from a quantitative standpoint
even in its early stages is quite impressive. It
is estimated that a complete sweep of six slides
at 20 RPM takes approximately one hour. Using
the conservative estimate of 100 usable cells for
six slides, the various machine operations will
allow complete analysis of 200 cells per day. A
similar completely automated system is also being
developed by Rutovitz et al.[31] For a more detailed discussion of the various automated methods of
karyotype analysis, the reader is referred to a
Symposium on Human Population Cytogenetics.[32]
Obviously, true cytogenetic monitoring on a population basis is dependent upon greatly expanded
facilities for chromosome analysis. It is equally obvious that machine applications to the problem are the only answer. In spite of those difficulties still to be overcome, the development
of automatic processing has made impressive
strides in the last several years. This progress
is continuing and hopefully, within a decade,
computerized karyotyping will be a routine pro-

cedure.

TYPES OF MONITORING

As indicated above, two types of cytogenetic monitoring are applicable to man. Screening for abnormal karyotypes within an exposed population has already yielded a reasonable body of data on the incidence of various abnormalities of chromosome number and structure in several human populations. Increases in karyotypic abnormalities would indirectly reflect germ cell effects, either on the process of meiotic cell division or on the chromosomes themselves.

Alternatively, or in addition, we may examine large numbers of cells in exposed persons for the presence of induced aberrations, presuming that an increased frequency of aberration-containing cells represents the effects of "chromosomolytic" agents. Let us consider the feasibility of these two approaches, and attempt to assess the likelihood that either of them will enlighten us on the exposure of human populations to potential environmental mutagens.

THE F_1 GENERATION

Transmissible abnormalities of chromosome number are generally viewed in man as arising from meiotic nondisjunction.[33] To date, no agent in man's environment has been definitively established as capable of affecting nondisjunctional evidence of induced chromosomal rearrangements in germ cells being transmitted to the F_1 generation. This does not suggest that such transmission does not occur. We know that for radiation exposure, for example, it must. But, the magnitude of any increase in abnormalities of chromosome number or structure in the F_1 generation is generally so small as to escape our detection. Loss of chromosomally altered germ cells; selection against such cells during fertilization; and undetected fetal wastage all mitigate against the production of viable, chromosomally abnormal offspring.

The cytogenetic study of the F_1 generation in Hiroshima and Nagasaki indicates the scope of the problem. The question was, and still is, whether the gamma and neutron radiations of the atomic bombs increased nondisjunction, or induced chromosomal rearrangements, in the parental germ cell. A pilot study of 128 members of the F_1 generation, all of whom had at least one parent exposed to over 100 rad, revealed no abnormalities which could reasonably be attributed to parental A-bomb exposure.[34] This enabled us to say, with 95 per cent confidence, that the frequency of numerical aberrations or of structural alterations of the germ cell chromosomes, will be seen in less than 2.5 per cent of examined subjects.

This is a situation in which the agent in question is a known, and well-established, chromosomal mutagen. Further, the exposure dose estimates are high. The anticipated low frequency of detectable abnormalities means that thousands of cases will have to be investigated in order to detect significant differences between controls and the F_1 study group. Two complicating factors are the relatively high frequencies of a) persons with major chromosomal anomalies in the general population-0.5%, and b) the 2.0 - 4.0% of structural heterozygotes in most populations, i.e., persons with one structurally-altered member of a pair of homologous chromosomes, present in all cells, and often only detectable on formal karyotype analysis.[35,36] To determine, then, whether even a recognized chromosomal mutagen, in high doses, can increase nondisjunction or produce meiotic chromosome damage in man is no small task.

The application of automated computer techniques to an F_1-type study seems clearly desirable, and just about as feasible. As described above, the technology of several groups working on computer analysis of human chromosomes appears capable of providing highly acceptable, graphic representation of the human karyotype, obtained from 35 mm. film of metaphase spreads.[37,38] The cost per metaphase will gradually be reduced with time, as the research and development phase of this work gives way to its application.

While we do have good data on the frequency of occurrence of certain chromosomal aberrations, our cataloging is far from complete. For example, the estimates of XYY incidence in non-institutionalized males vary from 1 in 500 to 1 in 2,000.[39,40] It may be advisable for us to do chromosome analysis on all newly-born infants, once the computer technology is ready for large-scale population studies. This would serve not only to identify chromosomally abnormal persons, many of whom now go undetected until puberty; it would also give us firm data on the comparative incidence of various types of abnormalities between populations, and on the changing incidence of time within a particular population. We urge this as one approach to monitoring human populations for the effects of physical and chemical agents on future generations.

SOMATIC CELL ABERRATIONS

While we have little direct evidence that somatic cell chromosome damage in the occasional cell has any clinical significance whatsoever, recent evidence has provided some insight into the biological behavior of chromosomally altered cells in vitro. The evidence on the cellular level, coupled with that which has been generated over many years on the population level, enables us to come to grips, in a tentative way, with the possible implications of induced chromosomal damage in somatic cells.

Our thesis here will be that chromosomolytic agents ought to be identified and avoided where possible, because in most organisms induced chromosomal mutations, as induced point mutations, tend to be deleterious. Let us briefly examine first, some of the epidemiologic evidence on chromosomal mutagens in human populations; and secondly, consider the evidence that cells with aberrations may be biologically different from chromosomally normal cells.

It is safe to point out at this stage of our information-gathering that groups of individuals that have been exposed to chromosomolytic agents, or that have an increased incidence of breaks on a "congenital" basis, tend to have more neoplastic disease than those not so exposed. The data from irradiated human populations is here again the most conclusive. Whether one considers acute, external radiation exposure, as in the case of the X-irradiated ankylosing spondylitics[41] or the gamma and neutron exposed A-bomb survivors,[42] or the exposure of persons to internal emitters, such as Ra^{226} and thorotrast,[43,44] the evidence is overwhelming that not only do these people have complex chromosome-type aberrations, but they also have increased incidences of various types of tumors.

For example: the X-ray treated ankylosing spondylitics demonstrated significant increases in exchange-type chromosomal rearrangements and a clear increase in the incidence of leukemia.

The A-bomb exposed survivors of Hiroshima and Nagasaki are now, and have been, studied extensively, and the presence of detectable aberrations in approximately 50% of all persons exposed to over 100 rad 25 years ago is convincing evidence of persistent effects from the ionizing radiations of the A-bomb in that group.[45] Leukemia and thyroid carcinoma are well established radiation effects in those populations.[46]

The radium dial painters illustrate the association between radiation exposure from an internal emitter and malignant disease,[47] with chromosomal aberrations of the various types being found in the lymphocytes of persons with high body burdens of Ra[226].[48] The development of osteogenic sarcomas in persons with high residual levels of this bone-seeking isotope has been amply described, and there appears to be a higher proportion of chromosomal aberrations in those individuals with higher body burdens. Similarly, thorotrast has been shown to be related to the development of liver tumors, and to the presence of increased frequencies of exchange-type chromosome aberrations.[49]

In each of these four instances of radiation-exposed populations, there has been an approximate dose-cytogenetic response curve, i.e., the frequency of residual chromosomal aberrations is directly proportional to the estimated radiation dose. Further, in Hiroshima and Nagasaki, where there is a sufficiently large exposed population to enable us to comment meaningfully on tumor incidence, both leukemia and thyroid carcinoma seem to demonstrate, in a more general way, this same dose-response relationship.

Thus, one criterion for determination of the chromosomal mutability of an environmental agent ought perhaps to be the demonstration, at least within some reasonable dose range, of a dose-cytogenetic response curve, whether in vivo or in vitro. At some time soon, other objective criteria will have to be established for the testing of drugs (and viruses) before they are labelled as chromosomal mutagens. It is safe to say that at the present time, ionizing radiation is really the only agent which can justify large-scale population surveys.

And yet, concern about the significance of induced structural aberrations in somatic cells is necessary. Evidence from in vitro studies of aberration-containing cell populations, specifically the viral-induced transformation studies, indicate that chromosomally abnormal cells may be peculiarly susceptible to infection and transformation by oncogenic virus.

The early experiments of Todaro and Green demonstrated that it is the rare, mammalian fibroblast that transforms in culture under the influence of simian virus 40 (SV 40). But, if cells from persons with abnormalities of the karyotype, such as trisomy 21, or with a high degree of chromosomal breakage, as in Fanconi's anemia or Bloom's syndrome, are exposed to SV 40, the frequency of mutant, transformed colonies increases ten to twenty-fold. The fibroblasts lose contact inhibition and undergo a change in their colonial growth appearance.

Thus, the relationship between induced chromosomal aberrations in somatic cells, the increased incidence of tumors in persons with such aberrations, and the increased susceptibility of such cells in vitro to viral-induced transformation, is becoming well established. What is not, of course, established, is how these three relate. Recent evidence from Paton and Allison[52] suggest that many physical and chemical agents may have a common pathway by which they produce chromosomal abnormality. Deoxyribonuclease of lysosomal

origin appears to be capable of inducing chromosome damage, and these workers suggest that
damage to lysosomes, of whatever cause, may produce release of endogenous DNAse, with resultant
digestion of chromosomal nucleoprotein. These
observations have not been confirmed by other
workers.[53] Nonetheless, it is reasonable to consider the possible susceptibility of mutant cells
to oncogenic viruses.

While it is clearly desirable, then, to minimize human exposure to agents which are known to
induce chromosomal breakage, we ought not to
draw unwarranted assumptions about the clinical
significance of these aberrations. Even if it
can be established that an agent is chromosomolytic (a not very easy task), we ought not to
equate that action with carcinogenesis, or even
with mutagenesis.

In summary, efforts must be made to determine
the biological and clinical significance of
induced aberrations rather than to continue to
expand, in an apparently unsystematic fashion and
with ill-defined criteria, the seemingly unending
list of those agents which damage human chromosomes.

REFERENCES

1. Crow JF: Human Population Monitoring,
Methods for Detecting Chemical Mutagens. Edited
by A. Hollaender, Plenum Press (in press), 1970.

2. Revell SH: Chromosome breakage by X-ray
and radiomimetic substances in Vicia, Symposium
on chromosome breakage. Heredity (Suppl.) 6:107-
124, 1953.

3. Lea DE: Actions of Radiations on Living
Cells, Univ. Press, Cambridge, England. Second
edition. 1955.

4. Kihlman BA: Chemical aspects of chromosome breakage, Adv. Genet. 10:1-51, 1961.

5. Kihlman BA: Actions of chemicals on dividing cells. Prentice-Hall Inc. Englewood Cliffs, New Jersey. 1966.

6. Cohen MM, Shaw MW: The specific effects of viruses and antimetabolites on mammalian chromosomes. The Chromosome: structural and function aspects. In Vitro 1:50-66. Edited by C. Dawe, Waverly Press, Baltimore, Maryland. 1965.

7. Osterlag W: Chemisches Mutagenese in Menschlichen Zellen in Kultur. Abhandlugen der Mathematische-Naturewissenschaftlichen Klasse 1:1-24, 1966.

8. Cohen MM, Hirschhorn R, Freeman AI: Mechanisms of chemically induced chromosome abnormalities, Genetic Concepts and Neoplasia. 23rd Ann. Symp. on Fund. Cancer Res. Williams and Wilkins, Balto., Md. 228-255, 1970.

9. Epstein SS, Shafner H: Chemical mutagens in the human environment. Nature 219:385-387.

10. Legatar MS: personal communication.

11. Cohen MM, Hirschhorn K: Cytogenetic studies in animals, Methods for Detecting Chemical Mutagens. Edited by A. Hollaender, Plenum Press (in press) 1970.

12. Bender MA, Gooch PC: Types and rates of X-ray induced chromosome aberrations in human blood irradiated in vitro. Proc. Nat. Acad. Sci. (Washington) 48:522-532, 1962.

13. Court-Brown WM, Buckton KE, McLean AS: Quantitative studies of chromosome aberrations in man following acute and chronic exposure to X-rays and gamma rays. Lancet i:1239-1241. 1965.

14. Bender MA, Gooch PC: Somatic chromosome aberrations induced by human whole body irradiation: "Recuplex" criticality accident. Radiation Res. 29:568-582. 1966.

15. Ostergren G, Wakonig T: True or apparent subchromatid breakage and the induction of labile states in cytological loci. Bot. Nat. 315-375. 1954.

16. Revell SH: A new hypothesis for "chromatid" changes. Proc. Radiol. Symp. Edited by Z.M. Bacq and P. Alexander, Butterworth's, London, England, 1955.

17. Revell SH: The accurate estimation of chromatid breakage and its relevance to a new interpretation of chromatid aberrations induced by ionizing radiation. Proc. Royal Soc. Lond. (Ser.B). 150:563-589. 1959.

18. Evans HJ: Chromosome aberrations induced by ionizing radiations. Int. Rev. Cytol. 13: 221-231, 1962.

19. Court-Brown WM, Jacobs PA, Buckton KE, et al: Chromosome studies on adults. Eugenics Lab. Memoirs XLII. Cambridge University Press, London England, 1966.

20. Hirschhorn K, Cohen MM: Induced chromosomal aberrations with special reference to man. Comparative Mammalian Cytogenetics Edited by K. Benirschke, Springer-Verlag, New York, New York 49-67. 1969.

21. Ferguson-Smith MA, Ferguson-Smith ME, Ellis PM, et al: The sites and relative frequencies of secondary constrictions in human somatic chromosomes. Cytogenetics 1:325-343, 1962.

22. Palmer CG, Funderbuck S: Secondary constrictions in human chromosomes. Cytogenetics 4:261-276, 1965.

23. Brinkley BR: Ultrastructural aspects of chromosome damage, Genetic Concepts and Neoplasia, 23rd Ann. Symp. on Fund. Cancer Res. Williams and Wilkins, Baltimore, Maryland. 1970.

24. Bartlett MS: Some examples of statistical methods of research in agriculture and applied

biology. Suppl. J. Roy. Stat. Soc. 4:137-170, 1937.

25. Gossett WS: The probable of a mean. Biometrika 6:1-25, 1908.

26. Fisher RA: Statistical methods for research workers. Oliver and Boyd, Edinburg, England, 1950.

27. Stevens WL: Accuracy of mutation rates. J. of Genetics 43:301-307, 1942.

28. Lubs HA, Ruddle FH: Applications of quantitative karyotypy to chromosome variation in 4400 consecutive newborns, Human Population Cytogenetics. Pfizer Medical monographs 5. Edited by PA Jacops, WH Price and P Law. Williams and Wilkins, Balto., Md. 119-142, 1969.

29. Bender MA, Kastenbaum MA. Statistical analysis of the normal human karyotype. Am.J. Human Genet. 21:322-351. 1969.

30. Wald N, Ranshaw RW, Herron JH, et al: Progress on an automated system for cytogenetic analysis. Human Population Cytogenetics, Pfizer Medical Monographs 5, Edited by PA Jacobs, WH Price and P Law. William and Wilkins, Balto., Md. 264-280, 1969.

31. Rutovitz D, Cameron J, Farrow ASJ et al: Instrumentation and organization for chromosome measurement and karyotype analysis. Human Population Cytogenetics. Pfizer Medical Monographs 5. Edited by PA Jacobs, WH Price and P Law. Williams and Wilkins, Baltimore, Maryland, 281-296. 1969.

32. Human Population Cytogenetics. Pfizer Medical Monographs 5. Edited by PA Jacobs, WH Price and P Law. Williams and Wilkins, Baltimore, Maryland 281-296, 1969.

33. Stewart JSS: Mechanism of meiotic nondisjunction in man. Nature 187: 804-805, 1960.

34. Awa AA, Bloom AD, Yoshida MC, Neriishi S,

Archer PG: Cytogenetic study of the offspring of atom bomb survivors. Nature 218:367-368, 1968.

35. Lubs H, Ruddle F: Chromosomal abnormalities in the human population: Estimation of rates based on New Haven Newborn Study. Science 169: 495-497, 1970.

36. Court Brown WM, Buckton KE, Jacobs PA, Tough IM, Kuenssberg EV, Knox JDE: Eugenics Laboratory Memoir Series XLII. Cambridge University Press, Cambridge, 1966.

37. Bender MA, Kastenbaum MA: Statistical analysis of the normal human karyotype. Am. J. Human Genet. 21:322-351, 1969.

38. Rutovitz D: Automatic chromosome analysis. Br. Med. Bull. 24:260-267, 1968.

39. Jacobs PA, Price WH, Court Brown WM: Chromosome studies on men in a maximum security hospital. Ann. Hum. Genet. 31:339-358, 1968.

40. Ratcliffe SG, Mellville MM, Stewart AL, et al: Lancet i:121-122, 1970.

41. Buckton KE, Jacobs PA, Court Brown WM et al: A study of chromosome damage persisting after X-ray therapy for ankylosing spondylitis. Lancet ii:676-682, 1962.

42. Bloom AD, Nakagome Y, Awa AA, et al: Chromosome aberrations and malignant disease among A-bomb survivors. Am. J. Pub. Hlth. 60:641-644, 1970.

43. Vaughan J: Bone disease induced by radiation. Int. Rev. Exp. Pathol. 1:243-396, 1962.

44. Fischer P, Golob E, Kunze-Muehl E, et al: Chromosome aberrations in peripheral blood cells in man following chronic irradiation from internal deposits of thorotrast. Rad. Res. 29:505-515, 1966.

45. Bloom AD, Neriishi S, Kamada N, et al: Chromosome aberrations in leukocytes of older survivors of the atomic bombings of Hiroshima and Nagasaki. Lancet ii:802-805, 1967.

46. Sampson RJ, Key CR, Buncher CR, et al: Thyroid carcinoma in Hiroshima and Nagasaki. 1. Prevalence of thyroid carcinoma at autopsy. ABCC Technical Report 25-68, 1968.

47. Muller J, David A, Rejskova M, et al: Chronic occupational exposure to strontium-90 and radium-226. Lancet ii:129-131, 1961.

48. Boyd JT, Court Brown WM, Vennart J, et al: Chromosome studies on women formerly employed as luminus dial painters. Brit. Med. J. 1:377-382, 1966.

49. Fischer P, Golob E, Kunze-Mullner T: Chromosomal aberrations in thorium dioxide patients. Ann. N.Y. Acad. Sci. 145:759-766, 1967.

50. Black PH: The oncogenic DNA viruses: A review of in vitro transformation studies. Ann. Rev. Microbiol. 22:391-395, 1968.

51. Todaro GJ and Martin GM: Increased susceptibility of Down's syndrome fibroblasts to transformation by SV40. Proc. Soc. Exper. Biol. & Med. 124:1232-1236, 1967.

52. Paton GR, Allison AC: Chromosome breakage by deoxyribonuclease. Nature 227:707-708, 1970.

53. Cohen MM, Hirschhorn R: Lysosomal and non-lysosomal factors in chemically induced chromosome breakage. Exp. Cell Res. (in press).

DISCUSSION

DR. SMITH: In searching for evidence of fresh
mutation in the population there is certainly one
technique that can be easily utilized at the
phenotypic level of the patient and that is
noting the incidence rate of fresh genetic
dominant disorders such as Apert's syndrome or
true achondroplasia. Though we call such syndromes autosomal dominants we don't know if they
represent point mutations, duplications or
deficiencies but they do represent mutations in
the broader sense and should be monitored.

DR. WEITKAMP: With this method you lack the
clear relationship between gene and gene product
that you have, for instance, in monitoring for
protein changes directly.

DR. HOOK: Very astute diagnosticians would
have to be reporting these cases in any monitoring system relying upon outside ascertainment
to avoid confusion of overlapping syndromes such
as thanatophoric dwarfism and achondroplasia.

DR. SMITH: I visualize a system in which suspected cases in a region would all be reported to
one center. One individual very familiar with
the syndromes in question would then visit and
substantiate the diagnosis in each suspected case.
This would serve the additional purpose of providing the patient's physician with an accurate
diagnosis and enable more precise genetic coun-
selling. No more X-rays need be done than would

ordinarily be required for diagnostic purposes in
any event. Illegitimacy might well be less of a
problem in this type of monitoring than in monitoring protein changes.

Appendix I

The following report was the outcome of a workshop sponsored by the National Institute of Environmental Health Sciences in Bethesda, Maryland, on November 7-8, 1969. The workshop was called to consider methods of monitoring populations for the effects of mutagens in the environment and it's theme was thus pertinent to the same questions considered in this volume. H. Eldon Sutton was the chairman of the workshop. Other participants were Heinz W. Berendes, Barton Childs, Edward M. Cohard, James F. Crow, John H. Edwards, George B. Hutchison, Marvin Legator, Brian MacMahon, Robert W. Miller, James V. Neel, Margery W. Shaw and Niel Wald. Observers from various other government agencies also attended. The report was submitted to the Director of the sponsoring Institute, Dr. Paul Kotin, but should not be interpreted as the official policy of that Institute.

While the report overlaps with discussions presented elsewhere in this volume, it is presented to indicate somewhat different approaches to the problems and methods involved.

We thank Dr. H. Eldon Sutton, the National Institute of Environmental Health Sciences and the Wister Institute Press for allowing us to reprint it in these pages.

REPORT OF THE COMMITTEE FOR THE
STUDY OF MONITORING OF HUMAN MUTAGENESIS*

The protection of man's genetic heritage has become an issue of great importance. With the development of a technological society, and especially in the past few years, the environment in which human beings attempt to survive is radically different from that in which they evolved. Virtually every person in the United States is exposed daily to food additives, drugs and pollutants of water and air that were unknown prior to the present era. In most cases, the biological effects of these substances are poorly understood, and attempts to assess the effects have been hampered by lack of adequate methods of testing and by the very large numbers of substances which require testing.

One of the more obvious effects of an unusual chemical substance on an organism is toxicity. The generally adequate information on toxicity of common drugs and food additives fails to consider the hidden but potentially very deleterious effects leading to increased mutagenesis. Even where human beings are used as a final assessment

---

*Reprinted by permission of Wister Institute Press from Teratology, Volume 4, pp. 103-108, 1971.

of adverse effects, a particular drug is never
tested in all the situations (such as pregnancy)
and in all the combinations with other environmental agents that would occur, should it come in
to general use. The example of thalidomide is
sufficient to emphasize the potential disasters
inherent in present practices.

The problem of mutagenesis is especially of
concern because a dramatic increase in mutation
rate could well go unnoticed for years in the
absence of an effective system of surveillance.
Only a portion of new mutations would be expressed immediately or in the succeeding generation, and information on the incidence of
inherited disorders is grossly inadequate and
difficult to obtain. Yet, one cannot in good
conscience ignore the problem simply because much
of the effect is deferred to later generations.
It is important therefore to institute an effective program of surveillance to prevent insofar as
is possible deterioration of the human gene pool
through environmental agents.

The means of assessing mutagenicity have been
discussed in a number of conferences and reports.
The testing of specific compounds is fairly
straightforward in lower mammals and microbial
systems, and cultures of human cells promise to
provide additional test systems of special relevance to man. These and related tests are being
applied by a number of investigators and institutions, although the information so obtained is
still small in comparison to that desired. These
methods of testing will continue to be the primary means of assessing mutagenicity of specific
substances, and they should be strongly supported.
However, there is no substitute for direct observations on the human population, and the purpose
of this committee was to study the feasibility of

such observations. In making its recommendations, the committee did not attempt to assign a priority to monitoring of human mutagenesis as compared to other uses which might be made with the funds.

Several methods have been suggested as monitoring procedures. The following brief discussions summarize the consensus of the committee with respect to the prospects for meaningful information from the various approaches. It should be remembered that technical developments could radically change these prospects.

The Frequency of Sentinel Phenotypes

A conceptually simple means of noting a change in mutation rate, leading to a change in frequency of certain genes, would be to record the incidence over time of specific inherited disorders. In order to yield reliable information, such disorders should preferably be simple dominant traits with only a low incidence of phenocopies, expression should be reasonably uniform, the diagnosis should be simple to make, the condition should not be lethal in utero, it should be recognizable in relatives, affected persons should have low fertility and the condition should be observable at birth. Review of the dominantly inherited disorders of man yielded only a few approximating these requirements and only three, aniridia, achondroplasia and acrocephalosyndactyly (Apert's Syndrome) were considered to be of potential use in a monitoring program. Assuming a background mutation rate of 2×10^{-5} per locus per generation, the frequency of new mutations would be 1 in 25,000 births for each disorder, or about 1 in 8,000 for the three disorders considered as a group. To detect an increase in this figure within a reasonably short period following the increase would require screening several hundred thousand births per year, with the observations made more difficult by the existence of cases transmitted from the previous generation. Even with these disorders, the problems of changes of procedures for ascertainment and diagnosis and changes in illegitimacy rates are so large as to compromise the reliability of conclusions which might emerge from a survey. The extensive use of x-rays in diagnostic procedures for achondroplasia and acrocephalosyndactyly could add to the mutational load, achieving an effect opposite to that desired.

Genetic heterogeneity, with some cases dominant and some recessive, would be a particularly difficult effect to take into consideration. By way of compensation, accurate knowledge of the incidence of various malformations in general, and genetically caused disorders in particular, would be valuable apart from estimates of change in mutation rates. Thus one might well support collection of such data for other reasons, even though they do not promise strong information on mutagenesis. These arguments were developed primarily with respect to autosomal dominant disorders. The arguments apply also to autosomal and sex-liked recessives, but here there is the added complication of unknown effects in the heterozygotes, effects which either might increase or decrease estimates of mutation rates based on the frequency of affected persons.

Because of the problems associated with sentinel phenotypes, the committee considers this approach to provide limited information on mutagenesis. Surveillance of sentinel phenotypes is therefore not recommended. The development of improved diagnostic methods could change the outlook greatly, and it would seem worthwhile to re-examine this recommendation periodically.

Mutations in the Structures of Specific Proteins

A promising but unexploited measure of mutation rate is the frequency of new point mutations reflected in the frequency of new amino acid substitutions in specific proteins, such as transferrin, hemoglobin, albumin, ceruloplasmin and glucose-6-phosphate dehydrogenase. There is evidence suggesting that the total frequency of such events is of the order of 10^{-5} to 10^{-6} per protein per generation. If one screened 300,000 blood samples for 15 proteins, the expectation of approximately 90 new mutants would provide a good base against which to detect an increase in mutation rate.

As with other studies of human mutation, the problem of illegitimacy is significant in comparison to mutation rate. With a full battery of genetic markers, most illegitimacy can be detected. A difficulty of unknown proportions could arise in the case of products of X-linked genes, when X-chromosomal inactivation creates the possibility of an occasional heterozygous female showing a homozygous phenotype, with her male offspring being hemizygous for the unexpressed allele. Such "maternal exclusions" would require careful evaluation.

The collection of blood samples could be done conveniently by collecting cord blood at the time of delivery along with a sample of maternal blood. There is already sufficient experience with this in large scale surveys for other purposes to assure that it is workable and relatively inexpensive. The laboratory processing of such large numbers has not been attempted and much development would be necessary. Using existing manual techniques designed to handle small numbers of samples would require approximately 150 technicians to complete 15 systems on 300,000 samples in one year. The laboratory effort would, thus, cost close to one million dollars per year, since the major cost would be for personnel.

This extimate is based on each technician processing 100 samples for one protein system per day. It should be possible to increase greatly the productivity of a technician by devising special screening procedures, with automation of many of the steps. The first step in implementation would, therefore, be to support studies designed to increase the efficiency of operations. The cost could be made appreciably less.

This investigation would yield information bearing on several basic points of interest in genetics and would, therefore, attract the participation of scientists who might have limited interest in a program whose only yield would be mutation rate. For example, the mutant forms selected would be a valuable source of variant proteins with which to study structural and functional variations. Further, the distribution of mutations along the structural gene would provide information very useful in establishing intrinsic mutation rates of various codons, information which could help resolve major issues in population genetics.

An important benefit of a screening program would be identification at birth of a number of genetic defects which might otherwise go undetected until overt disease or a clinical crisis occurs. For example, Wilson's disease, sickle cell anemia, afibrinogenemia and glucose-6-phosphate dehydrogenase deficiency would be identified, providing useful information to those responsible for clinical care.

The committee recommends therefore that support be given to setting up a program of screening for mutations resulting in changes in structure of specific proteins. Initial support for such a program would be for pilot projects designed to increase the efficiency of large scale operations and decrease the cost per observation. Support should also be provided for research to expand the number of proteins useful in screening.

One theoretical possibility which is attractive is to measure the frequency of somatic mutations at specific loci. For example, the blood cells can be thought of as a clone with short generation time and with ample opportunity to accumulate mutants. It is conceivable that the accumulated mutations could be detected through screening procedures which identify the phenotypes of individual cells. This would permit an assessment of the cumulative mutation experience of single persons, a measure which would be of enormous value in identifying environmental agents contributing to mutagenesis. Thus this approach would be especially useful in the study of high risk groups -- individuals with industrial or medical exposure to potentially mutagenic agents -- where the numbers of persons involved are limited. Support for the development of the necessary methodology would seem to merit high priority.

Changes in Chromosome Structure and Number

An apparently sensitive genetic measure of environmental insult is the production of breaks and rearrangements of chromosomes. Recent estimates indicate that breaks are seen in one 1-5% of cells, the exact figure varying according to a variety of laboratory and other differences. The frequency of gross abnormalities in karyotypes of newborns is approximately 0.5%. Increases in either of these figures could be detected on a relatively small number of samples, a minimum of 10,000 being required for the studies of abnormalities of number

An estimate using the present manual methods for large scale screening suggests a cost of $50 - $75 per blood sample. Therefore, the laboratory cost for 10,000 samples would be $5,000. If interest were limited to breaks, the figure could be reduced. In the case of breaks, the opportunity to subdivide the population into subgroups with different histories of environmental exposure should be exploited, so that the numbers of samples should be kept large.

A promising development in the study of chromosomes is the development of automated systems. Present projections indicate that a fully automated system will be able to handle some 800,000 cells/year at a cost of three dollars per cell. This would be equivalent to 50,000 - 100,000 persons per year, or even more, depending on the number of cells per person. Substantial progress has been made in automation of chromosome analysis, and, in the long run, automation appears to offer many advantages over manual methods for mass screening programs. It is estimated that 2 - 3 million dollars per year would be required for two years from the present time to have an operational system. After that the cost would be 1 - 2 million per year.

The committee recommends that support be given as soon as possible to studies of the frequency of chromosomal abnormalities based on existing methodology. Support of large scale screening programs in several laboratories should provide much needed information on base lines in normal populations and should permit the examination of high-risk groups with identified exposure to special environmental agents. It would permit prospective studies and longitudinal studies on populations selected with minimal bias and might therefore serve as a base for many other investigations.

It may perhaps seem premature to attempt to set up at present a completely automated system. However, it must be remembered that a relatively long lead time is required for the acquisition of the necessary optomechanical and computer equipment. It is anticipated that a lag of one or more years would probably precede the two year developmental period mentioned above, while the fulfillment of the initial purchase orders is being awaited. Support should be given further development of such systems with the expectation that within several years they will be ready to assume a major role in monitoring of environmental effects.

The studies of mutations of specific proteins and of chromosomes fit well together, since both can be carried out on the same blood samples. Furthermore, collection of cord blood and maternal blood suggests collection of a sample of placenta also, since the biochemical investigation of placentae has become of considerable importance. The placenta is rich in enzymes and is the largest piece of tissue available with the fetal gentotype. A depository of these samples of maternal blood, cord blood and placenta would be a valuable resource for further studies. These specimens would permit the assay of many substances of environmental origin, such as insecticides and drugs, whose presence might be unsuspected at the time of collection. One might therefore have the opportunity to make associ-

ations between malformations and various agents
in a laboratory-based retrospective study.
Studies of the placenta could establish zygosity
in multiple births, providing a population invaluable for many other investigators.

The cost of the collection network necessary
for a study of protein and chromosomal abnormalities is difficult to estimate but could be considerable. If set up in a number of hospitals
with large maternity services, the cost could
well approach one million dollars per year. The
more the collection can be concentrated in major
obstetrical centers, the lower the cost.

The committee recommends that the possibilities
for central storage of specimens be investigated,
the samples to be made available for further
studies. The cost cannot be readily estimated
without further study, but the value of such a
resource would be very great.

Sex Ratio

In theory, exposure of parental germ cells to
mutagenic agents should alter the distribution of
males and females among the offspring. Several
large studies in man have been frustrated by
inconsistent results which render impossible any
simple explanation. Sex ratio appears to be an
exceedingly complex parameter.

The committee does not recommend special surveillance based on sex ratio. Such data will be
available for persons coming under surveillance
by other means, but it should be pursued only to
the extent that it is a by-product of other more
promising studies.

Asymmetry

Alterations of body form and surface features,
such as fingerprints, frequently result from

285

specific gene combinations and from abnormal chromosome constitution. If such conditions arise somatically, affecting only a portion of the body, one might expect a greater degree of asymmetry. The possibility arises therefore for assessing mutation through measures of asymmetry. Specific suggestions have been made that this be done by analysis of dermatoglyphics.

This approach is novel but requires considerably more development before a screening program is initiated. For example, whether or not known mosaics are indeed more asymmetric as predicted should be firmly established. The committee recommends that no attempts be made to start a screening program and that requests for development funds be judged on individual merit.

Relation to Studies of Carcinogenesis and Teratogenesis

This committee concerned itself primarily with studies of mutagenesis. This is certainly related in many instances to carcinogenesis and probably to teratogenesis. If the emphasis on environmental effects is considered, study of the three clearly is interrelated even though mechanisms may differ.

Advantage should be taken of all opportunities to coordinate study of mutagenesis with studies of these other phenomena. The populations to be studied and the samples to be collected will often be useful for the different purposes. Furthermore, the results of combined studies may well yield information not accessible in a more narrowly based study.

Conclusion

Of the possibilities considered, the cytogenetic and specific protein studies appear most promising, with priority for a smaller scale cytogenetic study using present methods. Such a study could serve as a pilot project, yielding information useful from the point of view of genetics and providing an opportunity to develop the protocols, methodology and current cost estimates necessary for the ultimate large scale program envisioned.

The ultimate goal of carrying out cytogenetic and biochemical studies on some 300,000 samples would be a large and expensive program. The estimates given here are some four million dollars per year, but this estimate is crude. Nevertheless, the studies outlined here would appear to be of great potential, both in the medical information produced and in the contributions to basic research. It is hoped therefore that the National Institute of Environmental Health Sciences will be able seriously to consider supporting the developmental phases of this program.

VI. CONCLUSION

OVERVIEW

Kurt Hirschhorn

I will make a few general comments and then summarize some of the special problems raised by several of the speakers and, perhaps, some they did not raise.

First of all, we have some confusion of terms, namely: mutagenesis, teratogenesis and carcinogenesis. It has become the fashion to use these three terms interchangeably. Just because an agent shows some of each of these effects, or just because certain parts of the population show a high correlation between these factors, it does not imply that the mechanisms are the same. They may well be, but we do not yet have any evidence that this is so. One should, therefore, look at each of these effects as a separate problem for monitoring and not try to generalize.

A second problem is that which has been loosely termed "confidentiality of data". Few people have specifically explained what they are going to do with the information they acquire during monitoring. Who receives this data? How much of it will be individually identified? What will be relevant to the individual who has been screened without, at the same time, releasing them in such a fashion that there is invasion of privacy? Inadequate confidentiality could ruin the entire project.

With Dr. Murphy's questions in mind, I will attempt to review some of the points that have been made. The questions I am referring to are: What are we monitoring? What is cause and effect?

How are we going to monitor? What can we do about
it and what should we do about it?

One of the principles that has come out of the
first sessions is that the closer to the time of
the teratogenic or mutagenic event we can monitor,
the better the result. If we are screening
pregnancies by amniocentesis the parents are
available earlier, are interested in the outcome
and more likely to be cooperative. So, in the
long run, this may, in fact, be the ideal time
for monitoring but certainly we are not yet prepared to do this on a large scale.

The question of monitoring embryos, as Dr. Shepard pointed out, involves an enormous number of
unknown selective factors. We are missing perhaps
the most important portion of this information
(the missed abortions) if it is to be used for
monitoring. I think it is an important study
from the point of view of human embryogenesis and
teratology but whether it can be either mathe-
matically or rationally called "monitoring" is
something that I think needs reconsideration.

The problem in J. Miller's technique is, as he
pointed out to us, information retrieval. In his
particular approach there is a bias related to
therapeutic abortions, there is the question of
missing the early spontaneous abortions, there is
the question of macerated fetuses and there is
the bias of the hospital. These are all problems
that make me doubtful whether this is a "monitoring" technique, that is, one which can give us
information from which we can generalize to a
whole population.

As Dr. Fraser pointed out, monitoring major
congenital malformations is obviously a useful
approach to the study of teratogenesis if major
malformations reflect the action of the teratogens. We must also distinguish between monitoring
for teratogenesis and monitoring for mutagenesis.

The mere fact that there is a genetic tendency to respond to a certain teratogenic insult with a specific malformation has no bearing on this. That genetic background is there anyway -- we are not really checking for new mutations in any sense of the word. We are checking for susceptibility, expressed as a threshold when exposed to certain teratogens. If we accept and recognize this limitation, I think such a study can be of value but let us not confuse it with monitoring mutagenesis.

Similarly, in Robert Miller's discussion of cancer surveillance in children, we come to the problem of possible confusion of carcinogenesis, mutagenesis and teratogenesis. Again, correlations do not necessarily mean cause and effect. These particular types of studies, therefore, must be designed to ask specific questions and not be made into a universal monitoring system to try to answer a variety of possibly unrelated questions.

The minor anomalies provide us with perhaps even more of a problem. First of all, they are common. The discussions by Smith and Hook on the question of minor anomalies have been useful and perhaps some of these can be introduced into monitoring systems but we are far from the criterion of looking for a primary gene defect. It would be an advantage in monitoring major defects if it were found that there are people who are susceptible and then when exposed to teratogenic agents will express this susceptibility. But, for minor defects (for instance, dermal ridge patterns) we have the problem of inherited variation. This is particularly true if there is reduced penetrance of such an inherited factor. We probably cannot look at a single, minor malformation and say that it is meaningful because we do not know the findings in the parents, i.e. whether this defect simply represents a gene or a set of genes that these parents carry. There are numerous examples of this. If one screens for broad thumbs and toes, one will confound the dominant gene for broad thumbs with a totally different, possibly genetically-determined set of symptoms called the Rubenstein-Taybi syndrome, and possibly with a variety of other related genes, which will confuse the meaning of the appearance of a minor malformation. Once again, teratogenesis and mutagenesis have to be carefully separated.

It may be true, as was suggested, that the presence of multiple anomalies in a new event may be far better than a single minor anomaly which may be nothing more than the expression of a gene which was reduced in expressivity in the previous generation.

The three papers concerning the use of vital records deal with what I feel is a valuable approach but I wonder how meaningful the current results are for monitoring. For example, the inadequate reporting listed by Banister is an important limiting factor. What's more, if we now make propaganda for more reporting, as was suggested by all three papers, we suddenly will get an apparent rise in rate. This has to be carefully sorted out. Further, once the propaganda is finished, the apparent rate will decline. This can severely damage this type of study. Again, as we mentioned, these studies must be done with careful attention to the problem of confidentiality and invasion of privacy.

The fact that Milham retrospectively could pick up the thalidomide and the rubella situation is interesting. The thalidomide conclusion relies, however, on only one number in his table, but it is significant. I wonder, however, about the

conclusion concerning rubella. While the reported rubella cases show a bell-shaped curve
with a peak in April of 1964 of 11,000 and sur-
rounded by March and May with 8,000 and 9,000
cases, some of the characteristics occur with
only a single month's peak. We would really
expect, however, several months of increase. The
observation of an increase thus may be just fortuitous or reflect a real rise in incidence.
Perhaps it is a combination of the two.

The report by Flynt on the Atlanta system seems
hopeful since it is project-oriented and this is
important in the early attempts of planning monitoring systems. One must ask specific questions,
otherwise I don't think we are going to get
specific answers.

Ebbin's report regarding the Los Angeles County
rubella vaccine experience is interesting but, as
he pointed out, a bit premature because of the
low number of cases that have been reported.

The biochemical discussions of Scheinberg,
Weitkamp and the comments by Sutton are addressed
to problems closer to the gene. It cannot be
stressed too strongly that Scheinberg's search is
predominantly for disease. His quantitative
methodology depends upon an abnormality, whereas
Weitkamp's approach is a search for an increase
in frequency of genes not dependent on medical
abnormalities or any kind of prenatal, post-natal
or any other selective factor. There is, however,
one example using the approach of Scheinberg that
could be considered from the latter point of
view. The detection of the carrier state for
Tay-Sachs disease can be done with a simple quantitative method which has the potential for being
automated with the fluorimetry that Scheinberg
described. The enzyme whose deficiency is
responsible for Tay-Sachs disease, hexosaminidase
A, represents a heat labile isozyme. If one runs

a sample through the machine with and without pre-heating, one can detect what proportion of the total hexosaminidase is A. As O'Brien has described, and as has been confirmed in my laboratory, the heterozygote for Tay-Sachs disease has a markedly reduced level of this particular enzyme. There is almost no overlap between the normal and the carrier. Here, then, we have a single gene effect close to the primary gene product, that we can detect by quantitative methodology. It is crucial, if we are going to do any kind of monitoring, to be able to monitor single gene changes and not the homozygous state for an abnormal gene.

As to Weitkamp's proposals, one can only comment upon these by summarizing his statements that the prospects currently are poor. The money, the manpower and the techniques are simply not available.

During discussion, Smith brought up the question of screening for dominant disorders. I have been hearing for the past ten years that we should be screening for achondroplastics to determine human mutation rate. I hear it a bit less now, but I think it is still worthwhile to discuss what the difficulties are with this type of study. There is, of course, the problem of phenocopies caused by recessive conditions. For example, thanatophoric dwarfism at birth, without adequate x-ray studies and without Smith's expertise can be easily mistaken for achondroplasia. No one knows about phenocopies caused by non-genetic phenomena and, after all, we cannot know whether something is a new mutation or a phenocopy until the proposed mutant has delivered an abnormal child with the same mutation. As Murphy pointed out to me, we must remember that these types of so-called dominants can be produced by multiple loci. The gene for the α-chain of hemoglobin

one of the best studied human proteins, may be
duplicated at least once in the genome. It is
even better established that there are at least
two copies of the gamma chain so that gamma chain
abnormalities could be caused by mutations at
either locus. Of course, one is so far away from
the primary gene product in the study of the dominant phenotypes that the problem is even worse.
If we could develop a marker for achondroplasia,
it would be an entirely different story, for then
we could eliminate the problem of decreased expressivity in a parent in whom we do not detect
the phenotype because of some internal or external environmental factor that is suppressing the
expression of the particular gene. For example,
there are many people who are called new mutants
for X-linked Duchenne's muscular dystrophy because one can't find cases in the rest of the
family and one finds normal creatine phosphokin-
ase levels in the mother. But this is becoming
less and less sure because as the mothers are
studied more carefully with electromyography and
muscle biopsy of electrically abnormal muscle,
more and more of them turn out to be heterozygous
for the gene.

As for the cytogenetic discussions, here again
one has to differentiate between two types of
screening. One is the screening of environmental
agents and the other is sceening for the effects
of such agents on populations. The approaches to
each are quite different. It goes without saying
that the methodology is an essential part of
either type of study. In terms of screening
populations for cytogenetic variation, I think we
can go beyond just looking for breakage. Recently, for example, in a six month period at
Mt. Sinai Hospital during which 2,000 children
were born, we found four babies with Trisomy 18.
This means one in 500 during that particular

period as opposed to the expected one in 10,000.
From this point of view, chromosome registries,
such as the one the Birth Defects Institute is
developing, may be rather useful but this is not
cytogenetic screening. Unless we do chromosome
studies on the other 2,000 newborns, we do not
know what else may have happened. Perhaps some
epidemiological expert ought to go into that population to see if, in fact, anything did happen.
However, we are a bit late because it is always
at least nine months after the event if these are
caused by meiotic nondisjunction. As to mitotic
nondisjunction, it is evident that chromosomes
which have a small morphological abnormality may
be more liable to mitotic nondisjuction. Thus
the presence of mitotic nondisjunction may be a
clue to chromosomal aberrations in the parents.
It must be stressed that the types of aberrations
discussed by Cohen and Bloom, which are particularly important, are the rearrangements, because
when we have rearrangements we also have the possibility of getting clones of abnormal cells.
Such stable aberrations, translocations, inversion
and so on, probably are the ones that are associated with increases in susceptibility to leukemia
rather than simple breaks. Therefore it is
crucial to attempt to differentiate those agents
which simply break chromosomes from those which
cause exchange figures and, potentially, stable
aberrations. Once again, we must remember that
we are looking for correlations with carcinogenesis and not necessarily with the mutagenesis or
teratogenesis.

Sutton's proposals for the use of somatic cell
genetics are exciting. It must be remembered, as
he implied, that loss of a detectable protein
marker is never as significant as a change from
one detectable type to another. A loss of A
can be due to a variety of metabolic factors but

an actual change of a gene product from A to B
is more likely to reflect a mutation.

There may be other types of somatic cell genetic
mutational systems. For example, a study that
Chessin did some time ago in my laboratory used
human diploid amnion cells in culture. He
selected from the primary trypsinized amnions
cells which were relatively resistant to polio
virus infection. These rare cells could be
cloned, then recloned and shown always to breed
true for polio resistance. In this type of
approach, the genetic stability of a marker is
extremely important.

The question that remains: which of Murphy's
questions have we answered? As to his first
question - "Why monitor?" - for mother and
country - what else can be said? As to the other
questions of how to monitor and what to monitor,
I am sure that the participants in this Symposium
have given each other and to all of us a number
of ideas that deserve following up, although we
cannot at this time tell which, if any, of the
particular suggestions will be the most successful ones.

Appendix II

STATEMENTS REGARDING THE CONFIDENTIALITY OF
RECORDS IN SURVEILLANCE AND REGISTRY PROGRAMS

DR. JAMES R. MILLER: Dr. Hirschhorn has raised
the question of confidentiality of data in a surveillance program, and pointed out that there has
been almost no comment on this important subject
during the course of the symposium. Since this
question constantly comes up in connection with
the British Columbia Registry for Handicapped
Children and Adults, I thought that a statement
on this matter might be useful.
First of all, I think it should be stated that
the concern of most people stems from the fact
that a Government agency maintains the records.
Although abuse or misuse of this information is
not implicit in a Government's collection and
maintenance of such data, it behooves the agency
concerned to build in guarantees. Second, critics
of such systems should realize that other record
keeping systems are accepted without comment
although the guarantees of confidentiality are
almost non-existant (e.g. hospital records). The
British Columbia Registry has one cardinal rule:
there is no contact between the Registry personnel and individuals (or their families) who are
registered. Any follow-up procedures are carried
out by the person or agency who did the original
registering. The fact that the Registry is part
of the Vital Statistics Branch of the Provincial
Government means that the information on file is
treated with the same respect given vital records
such as births, deaths, etc.
In addition, there is a provincial statute
which protects the individual who registers, the

the person who is being registered and anyone who uses the registry data, and guarantees that no registry material can be introduced into a court of law.

Although no one can guarantee complete confidentiality (anyone who deliberately sets out to obtain a specific piece of information will find a way) those who establish surveillance and registry systems, despite the best of motivations, should be concerned at all times about the possible abuse of the information which they possess.

DR. PHILIP BANISTER: Dr. Hirschhorn's question of confidentiality of records is a good one. Since we were involved in the follow-up of cases, I would like to point out that it was most important that the follow-up was done through the regular channels of the Province. There was no attempt whatsoever to make actual contact with individual patients, since this might suggest that there had been dispensation of names.

Both the operation of a registry and monitoring, which is a different process, run into the problems of follow-up of cases and the following of cohorts.

Now, in terms of monitoring or surveillance, if you use vital records there is a well established procedure to safeguard confidentiality. Anybody who has access to them has to usually declare or swear an oath that they will maintain confidentiality. If you are dealing in terms of follow-up of cases for provision of care then this should be the province of the reporting physician. He should be the one who is responsible for the confidentiality of the information.

SUBJECT INDEX

A

Abortion(s)
  incomplete, 48
  maternal history, 38
  registries of, 56
  seasonal trends, 52
  specimen rate, 39
  spontaneous, 37, 38, 43, 47, 56, 60,
      61, 64, 70, 72, 73, 76, 87
  therapeutic, 33, 37, 38, 43, 64, 70,
      73, 76
Acardiac monsters, 54
Achondroplasia, 63, 273, 278, 296, 297
Acid phosphatase, 220
Adactyly, 39
Adenosine deaminase, 219, 220
Adenylate kinase, 220
Afibrinogenemia, 281
Albumin, 214, 215, 221, 226, 280
Alkylating agents, 251
Amethopterin, 193
Amethopterin embryopathy, 180
Amniocentesis, 25-27
Amputation, congenital, 63
Anemias, *see also* specific diseases
  hereditary, 214
Anencephaly, 39, 53, 63, 85, 87, 88, 114,
      115, 125, 134
  clusters, 116
  racial differences, 90, 91
  rates, 87-91

seasonal trends, 88
sex ratio, 90, 91, 114
Aniridia, 278
Antibiotics, 251
Antigens, red cell, 224
α-1-Antitrypsin, 210, 214-216
Anus, imperforate, 125, 134
Apert's syndrome, 183, 273, 278
Asymmetry, 202, 285
Autoanalyzers, 210
Autopsy, fetal, 77
8-Azaguanine, 244

B

Backcrossing, 21
Birds, malformations in, 107
Birth certificates, 99, 100, 114, 115, 120,
      121, 144, 150
Birth defects
  clusters of, 157
  costs of monitoring, 157
Birth weight, low, 4
Blood
  fetal, 34
  umbilical cord, 26, 209, 280, 284
Blood group A, 239
Blood group O, 239
Bloom's syndrome, 255, 266
Bone cancer, 97, 98, 107
Brain cancer, 98

303

SUBJECT INDEX

M